Contents

£13.50

THE · BUSINESS · SIDE · · · CTICE

Making Sense of
Personnel Management

SALLY IRVINE and HILARY HAMAN

WITH A FOREWORD BY

NORMAN ELLIS

RADCLIFFE MEDICAL PRESS

OXFORD

British Library Cataloguing in Publication Data
A catalogue record for this book is available from the British Library

Phototypeset by Intype, London
Printed and bound in Great Britain by
T.J. Press (Padstow) Ltd, Padstow, Cornwall.

The Business Side of General Practice

Editorial Board

Foreword

PEOPLE are the most expensive part of any organization's budget; they are expensive in terms of money, time, environmental needs and social and emotional demands. If management is about getting things done through other people, then the way in which an organization handles its human resources is crucial to its success. As a consequence, personnel management as a profession has been an integral part of good management for decades. Its value has been recognized, not only through its professionalism and its professional institutions, but through the increasing range of literature available.

This book makes an important contribution to that literature by setting out how personnel management can contribute to general practice. It does this by identifying and describing key issues in general practice where personnel management can help.

General practice is an integral part of our health service because it is so people-centred, and depends upon partners and partnership relations, staff motivation, supervision and organization, and patient relationships and communication. Good personnel management, therefore, is vital to the effective delivery of patient care. In addition the emphasis on audit and performance appraisal, both of which involve looking at how people do their jobs, is being felt throughout general practice. The sensitivities that can arise within organizations such as general practices which are still predominantly male-led and female-resourced are potentially very great. These can be exacerbated by the fact that in general practice the owner/manager of the organization is rarely trained in management skills and techniques.

The authors of this book are experienced in both management generally and also in the more specific field of personnel management. Furthermore both have considerable knowledge of management requirements and problems. Case studies and examples used throughout are all drawn from their experience as consultants and advisers on management in general practice.

As doctors have become increasingly aware of their legal obligations and responsibilities, the need for this book has grown. Although it is not primarily a legal textbook, it can undoubtedly help to reduce the risk of appearing before an industrial tribunal.

Managing people well is not simply a matter of luck, common sense and goodwill. These factors may be important but there is no substitute for professional expertise in personnel management; it can be learnt, its rules can be followed, and its impact can make all the difference between success and failure. General practitioners ignore it at their peril. A failure to apply the principles of good personnel management can prevent a practice from delivering effectively high-quality patient care.

NORMAN ELLIS
February 1993

About the Authors

Sally Irvine

SALLY Irvine became the General Administrator of the Royal College of General Practitioners (RCGP) in 1983. Her earlier career was in local government, where her responsibilities and experiences included considerable management responsibilities in the education field and later in corporate development, managerial advice, support and consultancy.

As head of the College's permanent staff, she has had the opportunity of using her management skills both within the organization and in the wider context of general practice, where she is well respected by the many general practitioners and practice managers who have benefited from her services as a management consultant. She writes extensively for journals concerned with improving management in general practice, and co-edited the very successful volume *Making Sense of Audit* (Radcliffe Medical Press, 1991) with her husband Dr Donald Irvine. She is also co-author of four management videos produced by the Royal College of General Practitioners with the MSD Foundation. Most recently, the Royal College of General Practitioners published her book *Balancing Dreams and Discipline*, on management in general practice.

Sally Irvine is currently President of the Association of Health Centre and Practice Administrators.

Hilary Haman

Hilary Haman is a Fellow of the Institute of Personnel Management and Vice Chairman of the Institute of Management Consultants (Wales and the West Branch).

She has 14 years' experience of personnel management and has worked in the private and public sector, three years of which were spent as Head of Personnel Services for the Royal College of General Practitioners in London. Since 1990 she has worked as an independent management consultant designing and running management development courses and programmes for general practitioners and practice managers. She also provides consultancy advice to individual practices and has most recently acted as personnel adviser to the Royal College of General Practitioners.

She lives in Cardiff with her husband and three year old son.

Preface

ALL organizations depend for their success on the ability of the people who work within them to give of their best to each other. In general practice particularly, effective networking between people from different professions and with different skills and responsibilities depends upon an understanding of, and sensitivity to, each other's needs, motivations and abilities. General practice, however it develops, will always be a people-dependent service. The needs of those people, be they doctors, nurses, administrative or receptionist staff, must be satisfied and their potential developed to ensure that at all times patient care is being provided to the optimum level by a happy, fulfilled and stimulated team.

In most practices, personnel management is not given the importance it needs; it is frequently left to the practice manager or the part-time female partner.

This book provides a guide through the main steps in human resource management, starting with the recruitment and selection of new members of the team. The emphasis is clearly on employed staff but the interrelationships and interdependencies involved, and the skills and attitudes described, are as relevant for partnerships as they are for the more conventional manager/subordinate relationships. Indeed, as the strains on the partnership concept increase, many doctors may find the guidance just as relevant for the selection and induction of new partners.

It is stressed throughout the book that the whole area of employment and personnel management is now bound by legal constraints. A complete chapter is devoted to the contract of employment itself, to give a clear and relatively simple guide to the many – often unfamiliar – pitfalls.

Another very important but under-used step in the development of a useful and productive member of the practice team is the induction process. This provides an opportunity for an organization to ensure that it obtains maximum benefit from a new appointment as soon as possible. A sound induction lays the foundation for the effective motivation of all staff. This can often be achieved both through delegating responsibility and tasks appropriately, and by ensuring that the members of the team have the right skills to carry out those responsibilities to their own and the practice's satisfaction.

Once the right person has been selected and settled in the practice, the appraisal of performance follows. The chapter on introducing appraisal schemes contains advice and technical knowledge which may be new to many and which are as relevant for partnership appraisal as for staff.

The book concludes with chapters on the most difficult areas of personnel management: handling poor performance and unacceptable behaviour – areas which are increasingly important and relevant if the practice is to become effectively managed. The way forward is through the setting up of appropriate disciplinary procedures and machinery, and formal policies for dealing with the uncomfortable but inevitable situation where a post is found to be redundant.

Many of these issues are complicated and complex. Therefore they are illustrated throughout the book by a case study that traces a practice's development through the stages of personnel management. This, together with the many examples based on the authors' experiences, helps to translate those steps to the general practice setting.

We are very grateful to Brenda Sawyer, Vice-Chair and former Education Co-ordinator of the Association of Health Centre and Practice Administrators (AHCPA) and Practice Manager at Shirley Health Centre in Southampton, and to Dr Roger Chapman of 'The Surgery', Leighton Buzzard, Bedfordshire, for reading the case studies and examples and contributing many ideas to ensure their accuracy and verisimilitude. We are also very grateful to Martin Holman of Kennedys, Solicitors, of Ormskirk, Lancashire for reading Chapters 2, 7 and 8 and giving us the benefit of his advice on the legal aspects of employment law and to Carol Boroughs of London Zoo for her helpful and insightful observations on the text. Naturally, however, the content of the book at the end of the day remains the responsibility of the authors alone.

We would both like to acknowledge the support and help of our husbands, Donald and David, who sustained us patiently throughout the writing of this book, with many words of wise counsel and encouragement. Finally, we are both very grateful to Anne Nash and Leanne Lassman for not only providing the written word but also appearing to enjoy doing so.

SALLY IRVINE AND HILARY HAMAN

1 How to Recruit and Select the Right Staff

ALL organizations are social institutions where people come together to fulfil recognized roles and functions. The quality of the work performed by or through the people in the organization is the single major factor which differentiates the excellent from the merely good business, and the good from the mediocre (Hunt, 1990). General practices are no exception. Practices in the past were mainly small organizations, often with a tradition of employing the GP's wife as the receptionist/bookkeeper. Later these practices developed informal recruitment methods where the new recruit was often known to the doctors. Such methods of recruiting staff are fast becoming a matter of history. The increased sophistication of general practice, and the consequent demands of practice life on the skills and qualities required of staff, are now demanding that recruitment is no longer undertaken so casually.

This chapter addresses ways of reducing the risks of making bad appointments, by applying a well thought-out and skilful recruitment and selection procedure, and by looking at the role such a procedure plays in the wider management of an organization.

The importance of the recruitment process

Unless they are creating a completely new organization or department, managers usually have to manage the staff they inherit. Although the quality of the work performed by others is influenced by the skills of the manager, it is difficult nonetheless to change established attitudes held by those who have been in the business for some time. Thus the manager who is able to recruit personally selected colleagues has an opportunity to introduce different ways of working and raise the level of performance.

Recruiting and selecting the right staff is therefore crucial. It is an opportunity which is often under-used, however, and which often goes wrong, leading to considerable repercussions. Appointing an unsuitable applicant can cause distress to the practice and the individual concerned. No favours are being done to anybody, least of all the successful candidate, if the new appointee and the practice are not well matched (Irvine and Huntington, 1991). The recruitment and selection of staff is a management activity which is vulnerable to subjective feelings and hastily made decisions. Moreover there is now a considerable body of law which has to be observed throughout the whole process (Ellis, 1990).

Despite the popularity and growth of selection methods such as psychometric testing and assessment centres, very few employers employ staff without first meeting them. Indeed, part of all selection procedures involves a series of encounters (usually interviews) between the employer and the job applicant where inferences will be made by and about each other. Even though research evidence shows that interviews are not accurate predictors of the suitability of candidates, well conducted interviews are more accurate than poorly conducted ones (Fowler, 1991). The quality of the interviewing is crucial in reducing the risks of making a bad appointment.

However, although it is common practice to define the recruitment of new staff purely in terms of the recruitment interview, it is only one part of the recruitment and selection process. The success of the interview as a method of selecting the right candidate will be determined by the effectiveness of both the preparatory work beforehand and the post-interview procedures.

The vacancy

Reviewing the organization – is there a vacancy?

If a vacancy arises because someone has left the practice, it is essential not to assume that the vacancy needs filling or that it needs filling by a person similar to the one who has gone. No organization should remain static. The more an organization changes and develops, the more profound is the effect on the jobs of the people who work within it.

Practices are fast becoming acclimatized to the impact of external change and developments within the practice become necessary if such changes are to be managed effectively (Pringle et al., 1991). Change is also initiated from within the practice. The appointment of a new partner or a new practice manager, an emergency call which goes wrong or an inaccurate diagnosis which results in premature death are all examples of events which should stimulate the practice into looking at its procedures and protocols, including the work of practice staff.

The future also needs to be considered. A departure provides a good opportunity to review an organization's structure and climate. A vacancy may offer the practice the opportunity to employ a person with the skills and/or potential to help it achieve its long-term aims. The process will of itself concentrate the practice's mind on the answers to the strategic questions set out in Box 1.1.

Box 1.1: Strategic questions
- Why is the organization here?
- What business is it in?
- What are its policies?
- What does it intend to do to achieve that purpose?

Source: Irvine (1992)

Review and analysis at the earliest stages in recruitment are part of the central management functions of organizational diagnosis and development, and require as much care and attention as is given to the clinical needs of patients. The effectiveness of the selection interview depends on the quality of the early diagnostic work in the selection process.

CASE STUDY (1)

The four partners of John Stroot Health Centre had a single item on the agenda of their regular weekly lunchtime meeting – the filling of the practice manager vacancy. The practice had experienced two practice managers leaving within one year, and was now feeling very vulnerable.

The senior partner, Bill String, started the discussion by describing his ideal practice manager – someone just like their original practice manager, Doris Pond – who would stay with the practice, know about family medicine, get on with people and not upset others. His list did not include any reference to tasks, duties or responsibilities that he felt should be delegated to this manager. Bill thought that getting the right person was the most important step.

'Well,' said Stephen Wood, the youngest partner, 'I think the whole point is first to try to see what we need. We know we aim to stay a training practice, to build new premises in the next two years, and to become fundholders. We've agreed that we want to be at the leading edge of good quality practice, and we want to increase our income if possible. All that can't be achieved without good systems, good decision-making processes, good records, good information, accurate and appropriate data, happy well-motivated staff, and partners working openly and frankly together with the rest of the team. We're going to be very busy carrying out the clinical aims we have set. We need to buy in the best help we can afford to ensure the management of this practice can match our clinical expectations. If it doesn't, all the clinical skill in the world will not enable us to meet our goals.'

Another partner, Veronica Iron, supported him: 'Well, I think that someone with the skills and confidence to manage staff and us in a way that makes us all feel fulfilled and not bossed around would be ideal. He or she would contribute to our discussions, stimulate and introduce new ideas, streamline systems, ensure we have the right data at the right time, negotiate with other professionals on our behalf, and maximize our income by looking at the way we use resources.'

Bill shook his head. 'That sounds very much like a manager take-over to me. Where do we fit in? We do own the firm after all!'

'That's the point,' said Stephen, 'We're the managers too – we're simply saying that in the same way as we delegate nursing activities to those more equipped and skilled to nurse alongside and in partnership with us, so we need to buy in management expertise to help us to do our part a bit more effectively, as well as actually doing a lot of the management for us. I don't want to be involved with negotiating cost rent schemes or organizing staff rotas.'

Tom Cutter interjected: 'It does seem to me that this discussion has made it clear why Doris left us after 20 years, and more particularly why Ellen Lake only lasted six months. We all have different views on the job and tasks involved, how much a practice manager should do. I can't see that we can get further with this without knowing which aspects of the practice can only be managed by doctors, what sort of decisions only we can take, and then which of those we need help with and what that help should be. Then we can look at the rest of the practice activities and say that they are the responsibility of the practice manager alone. How the practice manager carries them out – either directly or through others – is up to him or her.'

As a result the partners argued out a rough division between those parts of the practice's organization over which they felt they should retain strict control, such as agreeing expenditure over £100 (Stephen fiercely argued that this should be £1000), the appointment and dismissal of all staff, the appointment of partners, approving and signing contracts, the use of clinical time, and the use and management of the treatment room. The concession from Bill was that all these could be reviewed when a new practice manager was in post.

Having thus clarified the direction and expectations of the partnership, it was possible to draw up a job description and person specification that met the practice's known needs for the present and foreseeable future.

The exit interview

The first person to talk to when a vacancy looms is the person who is leaving. Such a discussion is commonly called 'the exit interview'. Leavers are a valuable source of information, not only about the job they have been doing but also about the organization itself. The case study (2) shows how the John Street Health Centre dealt with getting the views of the retiring practice manager, both on the practice and on her possible successor.

It is important to make it clear to someone who is leaving that there is a genuine desire to learn what the practice is like for staff who work within it. When people leave an organization they are sometimes anxious about the references their current employer will give to their new employer, so, if possible the exit interview should be conducted after references have been sent. If exit interviews are not held for fear of what an employee will say about the people and managers in the practice, then a valuable opportunity to gain insights into the practice will be lost.

The exit interview may well identify tasks which are now obsolete, especially in organizations which are changing quickly. It may also reveal ways of distributing the work to other staff, in which case the person leaving need not be replaced. Whatever the outcome, it is important to conduct the interview sensitively and carefully, however informally. Otherwise, as in the case of Bill String and the John Street partners, there is a danger the wrong conclusions will be drawn.

CASE STUDY (2)

Ellen Lake's appointment had followed Doris Pond's decision to retire after 20 years with the practice, for the last 10 of which she had been the practice's manager. When Stephen Wood had joined the firm, with lots of ideas about what a practice manager could do for the practice, and when the partners began to talk about fundholding and moving to new premises, Doris asked to be allowed to retire early. When she did, Bill effectively conducted an exit interview with her but made little use of the information thus gleaned.

Over coffee one day, Bill asked Doris what the real reason was for her retirement. Doris explained that she had taken on the post of practice manager as something of a favour to the partners, but she was never really sure what they expected of her, beyond 'keeping the show on the road'. She had attended practice meetings to take notes, but not to join in the discussions nor in the decision-making. Her views and advice were rarely sought and therefore rarely given, although once or twice she felt that the practice had taken a wrong route because they had not asked the staff their views. She had major difficulties in carrying out the one role about which the partners had been explicit – supervising the staff. Because she had come from within the practice, she was expected to move from colleague to supervisor without much help or guidance. It had been a stressful time for Doris but thankfully the staff were very stable and reliable. No incidents had occurred that required disciplinary action but she felt that if there had been the partners would not have seen the problem coming, nor have supported her in dealing with it. She had therefore been very anxious for a lot of the 10 years she had been in post.

Bill was surprised at her views, made soothing noises and said that perhaps it was for the best that she was leaving. Obviously she was not able to cope. Doris was too loyal and demoralized to do more than agree. Bill then went on – with some lack of sensitivity – to ask Doris for her views on who her successor should be. Bill was sure they should come from within the practice again. Doris suggested that Ellen Lake, the present senior receptionist, who had knowledge both of the practice and of the Health Service, would be an ideal successor. Bill was pleased with this idea and sold it to Tom, who felt Ellen was sufficiently different from Doris in that she was very ambitious. Stephen and Veronica were less sure, but Ellen was appointed without interview, and the issues raised by Doris were not addressed.

Box 1.2: What to learn from an exit interview

1 The type of work
  - Was the work within or beyond this person's capacity?
  - Did they find the work interesting or dull?
  - Were they over- or under-worked?
  - Was the job too isolated or too social?

2 The level of responsibiliy
  - Did they feel comfortable with the level of responsibility of the job?
  - Did they have the authority and resources to fulfil their responsibilities?

3 The clarity of communications
  - Was the person clear as to their role in the practice?
  - Was their role clear to their colleagues?
  - Were lines of accountability clear or ambiguous?

4 The type of atmosphere
  - Did they find their colleagues friendly and supportive or competitive and unhelpful?
  - Is working in this organization personally stressful?
  - What is the person's views of the difficulties?

Creating a new job

It is sometimes necessary to create a new post without someone leaving, either because of a rise in the quantity of work or because of the development of a new type of work which cannot be done by existing staff. In such cases it is vital to analyse whether the new job is on a lower, similar or higher level than existing ones. A new post should always be discussed with existing staff, as this creates an atmosphere of opportunity. Offers of further training to enable staff to do the new tasks show how the practice values them. Appointing from within is discussed in greater detail below (*see* p. 16) and is referred to in the case study (2 and 3).

Job description and personal specification

Once the practice is clear about the type of vacancy, time needs to be spent on preparing two crucial documents – the job description and the personal specification. These documents help in writing the advertisement and selecting the short list, and are crucial in preparing, recording and conducting the recruitment interview. It is important to take into account at this stage what has been learned from the exit interview.

Job description

This describes the *main duties and responsibilities* of the post, and should be written before the personal specification, which describes the *type of person* needed to undertake those duties and responsibilities. It is all too easy to merge the two and immediately start thinking about the sort of person to employ before a full analysis and description of the job has taken place.

Writing an accurate job description is a prerequisite to deciding what sort of person the practice wishes to employ. Expectations should be clear at the outset without compromising the contractual obligations of the practice (*see* Chapter 2).

The importance of the job description in assessing training needs and appraising someone's performance is described later (*see* Chapters 5 and 6), but Box 1.3 sets out the essentials and Figure 1.1 gives a sample job description of a practice manager.

Box 1.3: The principal elements of a job description
The job description must contain:
- the job title
- the overall purpose of the job
- the role/person to whom the job holder will be accountable
- the main responsibilities and duties of the job including responsibilities for other people, materials, and money
- an indication of those with whom the job holder will work

Job title:	Practice manager
Accountable to:	The partners
Responsible for:	All non-medical staff of the practice; the practice nurses will be responsible to the practice manager for the non-clinical duties of their posts.
Terms of reference:	To assist the partners in the management of the practice in order to help develop the quality of its care of patients.
Main responsibilities:	
1	With the partners, identifying and preparing the practice's 5 year development plan.
2	With the practice's chairman, preparing the agenda for monthly partners' meetings, and providing policy and management advice at such meetings.
3	Organizing and chairing a weekly meeting of all practice members.

4   Having responsibility for the per-
         sonnel management of the practice.
         This will include:

         i)   the selection, supervision, training
              and development of reception and
              clerical staff
         ii) establishing a performance apprais-
              al scheme
         iii) drawing up and regularly reviewing
              written contracts of employment
         iv) ensuring that employment legis-
              lation is followed and good man-
              agement practice is adopted, includ-
              ing development of the practice's
              equal opportunities policy
         v)   with the exception of the practice
              nurses, operating the first stage of
              the practice's disciplinary proce-
              dures.

5   Assisting the partners in maximizing
         the practice's income and controlling
         expenditure. This will include ensuring
         that the practice makes all appropriate
         claims to the Family Health Services
         Authority   (FHSA)/Health   Board,
         monitoring expenditure so that value
         for money is obtained, reaching the
         targets set out in the 1990 Contract,
         salary and pension administration and
         control of petty cash.

6   Preparing a full set of practice
         accounts up to trial balance and
         liaising fully with the practice
         accountant.

7   Monitoring and evaluating the prac-
         tice's administrative procedures and
         processes.

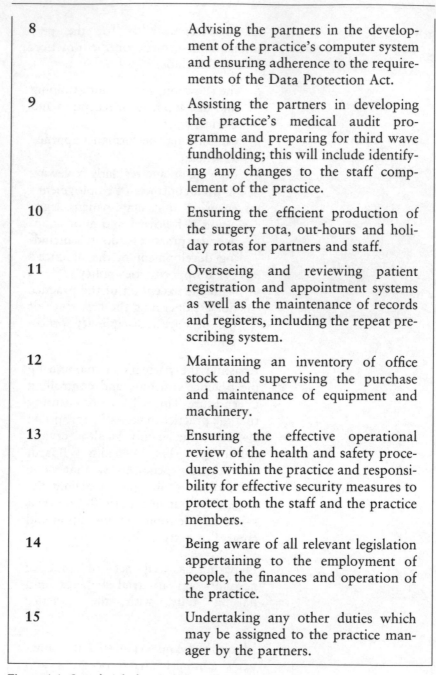

8	Advising the partners in the development of the practice's computer system and ensuring adherence to the requirements of the Data Protection Act.
9	Assisting the partners in developing the practice's medical audit programme and preparing for third wave fundholding; this will include identifying any changes to the staff complement of the practice.
10	Ensuring the efficient production of the surgery rota, out-hours and holiday rotas for partners and staff.
11	Overseeing and reviewing patient registration and appointment systems as well as the maintenance of records and registers, including the repeat prescribing system.
12	Maintaining an inventory of office stock and supervising the purchase and maintenance of equipment and machinery.
13	Ensuring the effective operational review of the health and safety procedures within the practice and responsibility for effective security measures to protect both the staff and the practice members.
14	Being aware of all relevant legislation appertaining to the employment of people, the finances and operation of the practice.
15	Undertaking any other duties which may be assigned to the practice manager by the partners.

Figure 1.1: Sample job description

Information on the terms and conditions of the post can be appended to the job description as further particulars. False or misleading information – such as any indication that the successful candidate will be promoted – can have legal as well as morale implications for the practice (*see* Chapter 3).

Writing a job description – collecting information

Writing a job description is time consuming and, depending on the complexity of the job, complicated. The first step is to collect the relevant information. There are a variety of methods. The choice is largely determined by the size of the practice and the complexity of the particular job. The five most usual are set out in Box 1.4.

Box 1.4: Methods of collecting information

- Observation: the process of seeing, listening and recording; good for simple jobs, but less effective for managerial or complex jobs.

- Interviewing: the most popular method of collecting information, particularly in small organizations; Chapters 1 and 6 cover this skill in detail.

- Questionnaire: preparing and designing questionnaires is an art in itself and not all job holders will place the same interpretation on questions.

- Group discussion: limited use as this method is only really effective if there are a number of people doing exactly the same job.

- Diary: the accuracy of this method depends wholly on the conscientiousness of the job holder.

Interviewing will probably be the analyst's main tool, but observation should be used to cross check.

The person doing the job is the most useful source of information and the job should be described as it is actually performed. However, employees can feel threatened when participating in writing up their job descriptions – any notion of some management plot needs to be quashed by explaining what is being done, how it is being done and the purpose underlying it. Confidence must be won and maintained.

The recording needs to be systematic. This involves a number of questions: what does the person do, how, and why?

The first question is vital and the second provides a useful check which can provide further detail. The third question provides a context within which the facts can be placed, and can prevent a misunderstanding of the real nature of the job. The very final question in any recording should always be: 'Do you ever do anything else in addition to the duties you have described (or which I have observed)?'

Accuracy, clarity and conciseness are essential in writing the job description. The job should be divided into its various tasks and it is helpful to record them either in order of priority or chronologically, as appropriate.

The 'what' and the 'how'

It is useful to begin each sentence in the job description with a verb and to strike a balance between accuracy and unnecessary detail. Each sentence can be regarded as a statement of what the person does together with a more detailed description of how it is done.

For example, health and safety may be the practice manager's responsibility. In the job description this could be described as follows:

'To ensure, as far as is practicably possible, that the practice follows the Health and Safety at Work Act 1974. This involves regular monitoring of the safety of the practice and ensuring that all staff are fully trained in their health and safety responsibilities.'

Responsibility and action

It is important to distinguish between activities and responsibilities. For example, the senior receptionist may be responsible for ensuring that the holiday rotas are done but she may delegate this task to another person. This would be described as:

'To ensure that the holiday rotas for the partners are drawn up and agreed.'

On the other hand, she may actually do the task herself, and in that case the statement would omit the word 'ensure' and simply read:

'To draw up and agree the holiday rotas of the partners.'

Layout

There is no ideal layout for a job description. The content and complexity of the description will be determined by the job itself and the purpose for which it is being used. For example, a job description designed to help fill a vacancy may include the main terms and conditions of employment. One designed purely to analyse the job in order to identify training needs and design a training programme (*see* Chapter 5) will probably have more detail for each main task but would omit the terms and conditions.

Personal specification

The personal specification is the document which translates the job description into a profile of the person required to do the job. It lists the qualifications, level of education, the duration and areas of work experience that the successful candidate will need, as well as any special aptitudes and personal qualities necessary. These factors need to be split into those which are essential for the successful delivery of the job and those which are only desirable.

Any factors listed in the personal specification need to be relevant to the job and not a reflection of traditional practices which may operate to the disadvantage of women, men, married women, minorities, the disabled or older people (*see* Chapter 2). Attributes, experience, qualifications and so on defined as essential should be those required by the post holder to undertake the work to the standard expected by the practice, after of course appropriate induction training (*see* Chapter 3). Desirable attributes and experience are those which would be nice to have, but are not intrinsic to the performance of the job.

Figure 1.2 gives a sample personal specification for a practice manager.

	Essential	Desirable
Education	General education to A-level standard	First degree: AHCPA Diploma Postgrad. Diploma: IPM, DMS etc
Experience	3 years' management experience in the health service	5 years' experience in practice management
	5 years' experience in general management where a significant proportion of duties involve personnel-related issues	
	Ability to prepare accounts	Ability to prepare accounts up to trial balance
	Familiarity with organizing meetings	Familiarity with organizing and chairing meetings
	Ability to operate a computer system	Ability to develop a computer system
	Awareness of equal opportunity issues	Readiness to operate an equal opportunity policy
Aptitudes	Good communication skills, written skills, ability to draft correspondence, policy/procedure documents	
	Good oral communication skills, ability to give	

	presentations to groups of staff and to communicate effectively with all levels of people Well organized approach to administrative work Imaginative approach to solving problems	
Interests	Authentic interest in and commitment to the aims of the practice	Involvement in outside activities which involve team work and interaction with people on a social level
Personality	Acceptable to all team members Ability to work as a team member. Ability to work under pressure Self-confidence but not over-confidence Self-motivation, sensitivity to others and reliability	
Physical attributes	Good general health Neat and tidy appearance Clear speech	
Circumstances	Ability to work irregular hours as	

required dependent on work demands	
Ability to commence work within three months of job offer	

Figure 1.2: Sample personal specification for a practice manager

Seeking the person

Within the practice?

The opportunity of looking for potential candidates within an organiz-ation is frequently ignored, particularly when there is no appraisal system (*see* Chapter 6) and managers do not meet staff as individuals on a regular and formal basis. Many people grow while they are in an organization and need a new challenge. Even if the new post entails a lateral move, this might be welcome to someone who is looking for stimulus and wider experience.

However, if appointing from within is going to work, careful thought needs to be given to the appointment and recruitment process both before and after the interview. It is a mistake to view it as the easy option. For instance, if the appointment is not successful, then it is much more difficult to handle. Informing an external appointee that they have failed their probationary period, although unpleasant, is far easier than coping with a long-serving member of staff who proves unsuitable.

CASE STUDY (3)

The senior receptionist, Ellen Lake, was duly promoted within the practice to the post of practice manager. Ellen was very confident of her ability to take on a role that was undefined by the partners and with expectations of her that were both varied and not explicit.

The partners left Ellen to announce her promotion to the rest of the staff. The news was greeted with resentment by two members of staff who would have liked to apply for Doris's job, and fear by others who had not enjoyed being supervised by Ellen when she was senior receptionist.

Much to Bill String's consternation, Ellen immediately demanded that she participate in all partner meetings and be given control over the work of the two full-time practice nurses. She generally upset the rest of the staff by her bossy ways.

Her anxiety to 'make her mark' and show what she could do meant that within a month the longest-serving receptionist had indicated that she wished to retire, and one of the practice nurses, Sister Stone, was threatening to leave. The partners were irritated and puzzled but felt powerless. Bill talked to Ellen about taking things more slowly, but the others just kept out of her way. They tried to pacify the staff, especially the nurses, by talking to them about Ellen in private moments. Stephen, the youngest partner, was known to have told one reception-ist that she should report to him directly if Ellen upset her.

After two months the partners were forced to deal with the situation when a serious crisis occurred. Bill had told Ellen that she was responsible for staff, and she would be held accountable by the partners for the proper servicing of reception. Ellen had always thought that Doris (the previous practice manager) had not been firm enough over the hiring and firing of staff. She told Bill that she had found a suitable candidate for reception, whom she had already interviewed and promised the post without consulting the partners. She had not even consulted the new senior receptionist, Betty Waters, because Ellen felt that Betty was a partner appointee, put in to keep an eye on her.

The partners had a very difficult interview with Ellen where she made it clear that she felt the partners had not made their wishes explicit; she felt that she had been undermined and abandoned by them. They still treated her like the senior receptionist, as did the staff. The partners felt uncomfortable and backed down in the face of tears and recriminations.

Fortunately a post of office manager was advertised by a local solicitor's firm for which Ellen successfully applied. The partners breathed a sigh of relief and vowed to carry out a proper recruitment process next time.

There are several ways of minimizing the difficulties of appointing from within the organization. First, an internal candidate should only be considered *after* the job description and personal specification have been drawn up. Just because a person is efficient in their current post it is not safe to assume that they will be so in the new post. If the vacancy is a managerial position, it is important to be aware that being responsible for the work of others is very different from and more stressful than merely being responsible for one's own work. A good administrator does not necessarily make a good manager. Equally, people will take themselves out of the running if they are aware that the demands of the post and the qualities of the person needed to fill the post are beyond their capability. Consequently, circulating a comprehensive job description and personal specification will deter some staff from applying for the position.

Secondly, consideration should be given to the amount of time and money the practice will need to invest in the appointment. Probably the person will not have undertaken this type or level of work before and will require support, training and coaching. Making an internal appointment in the hope that the person will cope risks a major cause of stress for many people, particularly when they are promoted to positions beyond their potential.

Thirdly, it is important to follow the same procedures whether the applicant is internal or external. Unless the application is ridiculous, it is vital to interview existing staff, but a skilfully handled interview can help the applicant understand why they may not be appointed. It is important to ask internal candidates the same questions as an outsider, to seek evidence of appropriate experience, to present hypothetical situations for their views and so on. If they are not appointed, they should be aware through the questioning why they are not suitable for the post. A formal interview will also ensure that both parties are absolutely clear as to the expectations of the post and the support the new incumbent will be given.

Fourthly, internal appointments can cause resentment among the staff. News of an internal appointment should be clearly communicated by the partners or practice manager, and staff should be informed of the implications of this new appointment. This eases the way for the new appointee and stresses the importance of the post and the support they will be receiving from the partners and/or practice manager. The internal appointee must have the vigorous and open support of the practice's management, and any resentment must be dealt with firmly and quickly to avoid resentment from staff who were not considered for the post or who failed the interview.

Finally, if a practice promotes a receptionist to the position of practice manager, the partners need to be aware that moving from being 'one of the girls' to a supervisory position is not easy. Indeed, in any organization, asking an employee to start managing their peer group can be traumatic. Relationships may need to be renegotiated and the new practice manager will need overt and subtle support from the partners. Expectations should not be too high during the first few months and a programme of training will be needed (*see* Chapter 3).

Box 1.5 summarizes the rules and pitfalls of internal appointments.

Box 1.5: Do's and don'ts of internal appointments	
Do:	*Don't:*
write a job descripton and personal specification *before* considering an internal appointment	rush into offering the job
assess the cost to the practice – time, training, coaching	view an internal appointment as a cheap, easy alternative to an outside appointment
be aware that managing others is very different from merely managing yourself	underplay the skills required to manage
hold a formal interview	appoint on the basis of a casual meeting or 'chat'
provide training and support	leave the new appointee to sink or swim
inform everyone in the practice of the new appointment	let the person appointed spread the news
anticipate problems with other staff and deal with them promptly	let the new appointee cope alone with hostility, resentment etc
give vigorous support to the appointment	assume that staff are aware of the support the new appointee will receive from the partners and/or practice manager

Recruiting from outside

There are two principle ways of recruiting from outside. The first is the informal network, but this can cause problems if the person so identified does not turn out as expected and is a relative or friend of someone in the practice. The second way is through advertising, in which case it must be decided how widely to advertise, in what medium, and how much information to give.

A very succinct advertisement encourages people to phone for more information, and time spent answering the calls initially can save time and energy at the later stage of written applications because it deters unsuitable candidates. It is also an effective method of assessing a person's telephone manner – significant if the vacancy is for a receptionist. On the other hand, advertisements which contain little information can attract a large number of unsuitable candidates. The personal specification is an aid in the design of an advertisement. It should contain enough of the 'essential' factors to attract eligible candidates and deter unqualified ones. Listing 'desirable' factors is a little more difficult: too many, and eligible candidates may be deterred; not enough, and ideal applicants may not be attracted. Advertisements must not discriminate on the grounds of sex, marital status or race except where there is a genuine occupational qualification in specific circumstances as detailed in the Race Relations Act 1976 and Sex Discrimination Act 1975.

There is one further piece of legislation with which employers need to be familiar when recruiting staff. The Rehabilitation of Offenders Act 1974 enables a person, including a prospective employee, to conceal from any other persons details of past criminal convictions which have become 'spent' as defined by Section 4 of the Act. Failure to disclose 'spent' convictions is not proper grounds for dismissing an employee or for excluding a candidate from employment. There are however certain professions, such as medical practice and nursing, which are excluded from this right to conceal a 'spent' conviction. These exceptions are set out in the Rehabilitation of Offenders Act 1974 (Exceptions) (Amendment) Orders 1986. Job advertisements or application forms for recruitment to such professions usually include the requirement to disclose convictions, including 'spent' convictions.

Box 1.6 contains the relevant key and optional parts of any advertisement, and Figure 1.3 gives a sample advertisement for a practice manager.

Box 1.6: Parts of an advertisement

Key sections:
- name and address of the employer
- job title
- salary or parameters of salary grade (do not assume that everyone is familiar with points on the Whitley Scale)
- the terms of reference of the job

- a selection of the essential and desirable factors (the essentials should outnumber the desirables)
- location of the job
- major benefits, eg pension scheme/bonuses etc
- who to apply to
- manner of application – CV and letter/phone for application form etc
- closing date

Optional sections depending on the post and the organization:
- date of interview(s)
- special features, eg extensive travel involved
- promotion prospects (ensure this is accurate and contractually astute)
- number of referees needed on the application
- equal opportunities statement

WE NEED A PRACTICE MANAGER

Salary £20K–£25K

A Practice Manager is needed for a general medical practice consisting of five partners and caring for some 11,000 patients. We operate from purpose-built premises with a full complement of staff – nurses, receptionists, secretaries, cleaners. The practice is situated in a pleasant suburb and is currently preparing for fundholding status.

The Practice Manager's main terms of reference will be to assist the partners in the management of the practice in order to develop the quality of its care of patients. The successful candidate will combine tact and sensitivity with an ability to develop efficient systems of work and to lead and work within a multidisciplinary team.

A minimum of three years' management experience is required. Previous experience of general practice, whilst desirable, is not essential. Essential skills include those of personnel management, account keeping and knowledge and experience

of computers. Relevant professional qualifications are desirable.
The successful candidate will be able to demonstrate good
communication skills, both oral and written, and a commitment
to primary health care.

This is a demanding post which will involve working under
pressure and, on occasions, irregular hours. The practice is
committed to equal opportunities and developing all members
of the practice team, including performance review.

Appointment on the above salary range will be determined by
the experience of the post holder. Study leave is offered after the
probationary period as is membership of the practice's generous
contributory pension scheme.

Please telephone . . . . for an application form and further
particulars of the post. Closing date . . . . It is envisaged
that interviews will take place on . . . .

Figure 1.3: Sample advertisement

The applications

The information provided by applicants will depend on the way the
practice conveys the job and its requirements in an advertisement and
in any telephone or personal contacts; the method of application will
depend largely on the nature of the vacancy and the management
style of the practice. If large numbers of applicants are expected, an
application form will be useful to make comparisons between them
and to construct summary sheets on candidates. However, forms can
restrict self-expression (important if this is a quality to be tested)
whereas a letter leaves candidates to their own discretion. A combination of the two is usual; a section of the application form is left
blank for candidates to express their reasons for applying, what they
can bring to the post and so on.

If an application form is used, detailed personal information (including marital status, number of children and ethnic origin) should not

be requested unless it is directly relevant to the *specific requirements of the job*. For example, if the practice is monitoring discrimination in accordance with the recommendations of the Arbitration, Conciliation and Advisory Service (ACAS) Code of Practice for the Elimination of Discrimination on the Grounds of Sex and Marriage, and the Promotion of Equality of Opportunity in Employment (ACAS, 1985), then this should be fully explained to applicants. Similarly, it is only fair to applicants to state clearly whether references will be used and at what stage in the process they will be taken up. It is useful to include on the application form a section for identifying the person's sickness record over the previous two years.

Each application needs to be compared with the personal specification for the job. This is where the time spent preparing the personal specification pays dividends. It ensures that assessing applications for short-listing is based on objective criteria directly relevant to the needs of the job. It is also a quicker method of drawing up a short list than assessing each application against some form of subjective ideal. If, for example, the essential factors of the job include shorthand skills, any applicant without this skill can be automatically rejected. The application does not need to be studied further once this gap has been detected. Each application which meets the *essential* requirements of the post needs to be examined thoroughly for gaps in employment history, areas which have been glossed over, a high sickness record and contradictory information.

CASE STUDY (4)

When Ellen left, and after the partners' meeting described earlier in the case study (1), the partners decided to advertise the post. The advertisement was very explicit and as a result only 20 applications were received, of which two were completely unsuitable. Each of the four partners saw all the applications and drew up a long list of six names. To their delight, and the satisfaction of Veronica and Stephen especially, the same four of the six candidates appeared on all their lists. They agreed that these should be invited to visit the practice informally and meet the staff, to see the building and to decide if they still wished to go on with their application. They also agreed that another four of the remaining long-listed candidates were worth seeing informally as well. To prevent all four partners being tied up in this informal process, they each undertook to look after two visitors and report back. The visits took place over two weeks. They had not warned the staff beforehand, and consequently there was a lot of disruption and upset. As Tom wryly pointed out, when he had received the second angry complaint from a receptionist about being interrupted by these strange people wandering through reception, 'another little wrinkle to learn for next time!'

The partners met again, after all the long-listed candidates had visited the practice, to consider who should be interviewed. They all agreed that if possible there should only be four candidates, because all the partners wanted to be involved in the actual interview.

As a result of the informal visits the partners deleted three candidates straight away as not being suitable for one reason or another, usually because the partner who saw them did not feel that they were temperamentally suited. Another candidate rang up after the visit to say that he wished to withdraw because the environment was too claustrophobic, and he did not feel that the doctors would allow him enough responsibility. Bill admitted that he was the one who had shown him round, and that he had found it necessary to curb the candidate's expectations of the job!

They were thus left with four: three women and one man. Two were graduates and three had experience in the health service, although only one was an existing practice manager from a single-handed practice in the next town. One candidate came from an accountancy background, transferring from mainstream accountancy to the managerial side of the firm in which she had trained. All were appointable on paper, and all had impressed in varying degrees at the informal visits.

They were called for interview, and the unsuccessful candidates were told by letter that their applications were not being pursued.

The interview

Before the interview

Calling people for interview

Recruiting for a vacancy is an opportunity for the practice to promote its image in the community. All applications should be acknowledged and unsuccessful applicants informed of their failure either to be short-listed or, after interview, to be appointed. Prompt acknowledgements are an example of good practice and good public relations.

In the same way, people begin to gain an impression of the employing organization from written and telephone communication before they enter the premises. Successful candidates need to be given details of how to get there and the amount of time the interview process should take. It is important to ensure that they are expected by the staff and made welcome.

It is at this point in the process that references are often called. There are advantages and disadvantages in receiving references before the interview. The reference can give an indication of areas which need to be explored. However some applicants may request that references are not taken up unless they are short-listed or even offered the post. This may be because their present employer may not be aware that they are applying for a new post. Moreover it can prejudice the interview panel, both favourably and unfavourably. Calling for references after the interview, particularly telephone references, enables the new employer to check out the information given at the interview and is probably more effective.

People apply for jobs in confidence and applications should be treated as such. The circulation of papers should be restricted to those involved in the recruitment and selection process, and not passed round reception for comment!

Arranging the interview

Decisions need to be made about who in the practice will interview. Are they those whose opinion is most relevant to the task of selecting the right candidate for this particular job? Interviewing is expensive in time and energy so the number of people on the interview board needs to be commensurate with the nature of the job.

Having said that, interviewing alone is difficult. Gleaning and giving information, probing and questioning whilst simultaneously taking notes is well nigh impossible. At the other extreme, large panel interviews can be daunting for the candidate and make the process very lengthy. If more than three people wish to interview, it may be effective to ask the candidates to attend two sets of interviews. Investment in the time taken to reach these decisions pays dividends later.

Recording the interview

An assessment form such as set out in Figure 1.4 to record each interview can be helpful.

The qualities on the personal specification can be listed against a scoring system showing if they are met, partially met or not met. Parts of the assessment can be completed from candidates' applications and the remainder completed during or immediately after the interview.

The advantages of using such a form for each candidate are listed in Box 1.7.

VACANCY: ....   INTERVIEWERS: ....   DATE: ....

CANDIDATE: ....   TIME IN: ....

                                                        TIME OUT: ....

PERSONAL SPECIFICATION			ASSESSMENT			
Factor	Essential	Desirable	Not met	Partially met	Met	Comments
Education						
Qualifications/ training						
Experience						
Knowledge						
Skills						
Attributes						
Other						

Figure 1.4: Interview assessment form

Box 1.7: Advantages of an assessment form
- Prevents interviewers confusing the candidates.
- Enables – indeed encourages – the recording of information as the interview progresses.
- Helps identify individual discrepancies which can be explored in the interview.
- Provides a long-term record for evaluating the effectiveness of the practice's interviewing/selection techniques in the future.
- Is in accordance with the ACAS Codes of Practice on the elimination of sex and race discrimination in employment and it promotes equal opportunity procedures.
- Helps ensure that the assessments made about a candidate are objective and not subjective.

Briefing the interviewing group

Interviews are expensive. The quality of the preparation will influence the efficiency and effectiveness of the interview. It is vital therefore to allow time before interviews to make the sort of preparations listed in Box 1.8.

Box 1.8: Interview preparation
- Ensure that each member of the interviewing group has a clear understanding of the way the interview is to be conducted and of any special area of questioning assigned to them.
- Plan a logical pattern to cover the most important aspects including education and training; work experience; existing knowledge and skills; ambitions; aspirations and outside work interests.
- Devise ways of obtaining evidence of intelligence, resourcefulness, capacity to cope if under pressure, persistence, attitudes to clients if relevant, degree of sociability (depending on personal specification).
- Allocate time for the candidates to ask questions.
- Ensure that each member of the interviewing group

understands their legal obligations under the Sex and Race Discrimination Acts 1976 and 1975, the Rehabilitation of Offenders Act 1974 and the practice's equal opportunities policy, if one exists.
- Ensure that the interview concentrates on the candidates' weak areas as these are the areas to explore. It is easy to spend a lot of time at the start of the interview on non-essential areas, listening to the candidate elaborate on their successes, and then run out of time when deeper issues need probing.

Creating the right structure and climate for the interview

The purpose of the recruitment interview is *not* to select a candidate – it is to gather as much accurate and relevant information as possible which will allow you to select the right candidate *after* all the candidates have been interviewed. It is also to give sufficient information for the candidate to decide whether or not to pursue the job. This second purpose can be neglected. It is important that new staff are fully aware of the realities of the job and the main terms and conditions of employment. Box 1.9 lists the purposes in more detail.

Box 1.9: The purposes of an interview
- To get as much information about the candidate in order to make a judgement of their suitability for the job.
- To ensure that the candidate gets as much information as possible about the job in order to make their judgement of their suitability for it.
- To explore the potential match between this individual and the practice.

This book refers several times to the importance of interviewing, and describes four different types – recruitment, training needs (*see* Chapter 5), appraisal (*see* Chapter 6) and disciplinary (*see* Chapter 7). Each type has a slightly different purpose and these need to be clear before each type of interview begins.

Gathering authentic information about the candidate will be aided if the interviewee is helped to relax. Unless the job demands an extremely high tolerance of stress, it is difficult to argue for stress-interviewing techniques, which are often counterproductive and may give the candidate the impression that the practice is an aggressive place in which to work.

Box 1.10 gives tips to aid a relaxed interview.

Box 1.10: The relaxed interview
- Arrange the furniture. The balance of formality to informality can be conveyed by the arrangement of the chairs and tables. A low coffee table is best: it is non-threatening and does not create a barrier. All the chairs should be of the same height and ideally be comfortable easy chairs, rather than straight-backed office furniture.
- Have a plan for the division of labour among the interviewers and share this with the candidates at the beginning of the interview.
- Give the interviewee an idea as to how long the interview will last and the areas each interviewer will cover.
- Plan for giving candidates sufficient time to ask questions and to develop their answers to the interviewers.

The interview itself

Interviews should be started on time – the candidate's time is precious too! Keeping candidates waiting can increase their anxieties and gives the impression of inefficiency. All interviewees are potential ambassadors for the practice; badly handled, late-running interviews can damage the practice's reputation.

The crucial skills in interviewing candidates are questioning and listening skills. These skills are often assumed. Open-ended questions which allow the candidate to give more than mere 'yes' or 'no' answers do not come naturally to most people, even though doctors usually have more experience and practice in this area. A conscious effort needs to be made to ensure that the candidate is giving sufficient and accurate information to the interview panel. One of the interview panel, who at that time is not doing the questioning, needs to follow up on a glib, short answer or aside. This is another reason why solo interviewing should be discouraged. Appendix A gives some helpful examples of different types of questioning.

Box 1.11 summarizes what to do and not to do when interviewing for recruitment.

Box 1.11: Do's and don'ts of interviewing	
Do:	*Don't:*
plan the interview	start the interview unprepared
establish an easy and informal relationship	plunge too quickly into demanding questions
encourage the candidate to talk	ask leading questions
cover the ground as planned	jump to conclusions on inadequate evidence
probe where necessary	pay too much attention to isolated strengths or weaknesses
analyse career and interests to reveal strengths, weaknesses, patterns of behaviour	allow the candidate to gloss over important facts
maintain control over the direction and time taken by the interview	talk too much

Questions which could be construed as discriminatory should be avoided. This includes questions on children, child-care arrangements and the geographical stability of the spouse's job. If tempted to approach these areas, then consider for example if an applicant's personal circumstances are really relevant, or whether having children or not makes for a more efficient receptionist/manager/nurse. Examining the reasons behind wishing to ask these types of questions will probably reveal concerns which lie in the areas of punctuality, reliability and stability. These are the issues to address in the interview, rather than the applicant's personal circumstances. Asking such discriminatory questions to all the candidates, even if all the candidates are married women with children, can still be in breach of anti-discriminatory legislation. Asking personal questions not directly relevant to the post is a dangerous practice, as many employers who have found themselves in front of an industrial tribunal can testify (Ellis, 1992).

Box 1.12 gives some ideas on the areas to cover in a selection interview.

Box 1.12: Points to consider at interview
- Why is the candidate interested in this vacancy?
- What is their reason for leaving their present employment?
- What is the depth of their interest in this job, ie:
    - do they show evidence of careful study of the documents supplied?
    - have they obtained any further information?
    - do they ask pertinent questions if given the opportunity to do so?
- Why do they feel they are the appropriate person for the job?
- Do they admit to any limitations/weaknesses in relation to the job?
- If so, how do they view these?
- Are their manners and speech likely to be acceptable to the practice?
- Would their attitude to work and to authority and to colleagues make them an acceptable member of the team with whom they would be working?
- Can you be reasonably sure that the behaviour you have seen at interview is natural and not assumed?
- If the job requires contact with the public, some of whom are often anxious and aggravated, is their personality such that they would be able to handle this and give a good impression of the organization?
- Would they be willing to accept the job if offered?
- When would they be able to commence duties?

CASE STUDY (5)

The interviews for the new practice manager were held on Saturday morning, with all partners present, although Veronica was half an hour late because she had forgotten to take account of the heavy weekend traffic. They had toyed with starting without her, but Tom was particularly insistent that they all waited. This put some time pressure on them as Bill had a family commitment at 2.00 p.m.

Bill chaired the interviews and took too long in introducing everyone. They had allowed 30 minutes per candidate but soon found that they were running over time, spending nearly an hour on each. Because of the delay at the start and because they had no kind of assessment form, they had not really organized who was going to cover what in the interview, and so no one was deputed to check career and health details. As a result they missed the fact that one candidate had a career break of one year because she had been dismissed for taking decisions beyond her competence, and had a period of unemployment as a result.

By and large the partners (apart from Bill) used open rather than closed questions, and indeed they got better at encouraging the candidates to talk freely, another reason the interviews took longer than they planned!

Selecting the successful applicant

Selecting the successful applicant should be done only after *all* candidates have been interviewed and each has been assessed in relation to the job description and personal specification. The interview assessment form is extremely useful at this point in the process. It provides the objective record of the candidate's history and interview performance against which the personal specification is compared. It is important at this stage to resist the temptation to compare candidates with each other. If not, the *best* candidate may only be the 'best of a bad lot'. Comparing candidates with each other is safe only when faced with more than one who could perform the job according to the criteria laid down in the personal specification.

Most research on interviewing demonstrates a pervasive tendency in interviewers to attribute qualities to others on the basis of physical appearance, and to do this within seconds of meeting them. Such attributes may turn out to be accurate, but more usually they are not. It is surprising how easily focusing on the post and its requirements can be forgotten when faced with a particularly personable and charming person. If such qualities are essential for the post, then the impact may not be so serious. If they are not, or if other qualities, skills, experience are as important, then the organization may lose by this distraction.

By paying close attention to the whole process of selection and not just the interview, the risks of snap judgements can be lessened. The assessment form (*see* Figure 1.4) ensures that the reasons why candidates succeeded or failed to get the job are recorded. This record is useful when later examining the accuracy and effectiveness of the recruitment and selection process and it may be needed should legal action be taken by a disgruntled candidate who feels they have been the subject of illegal discrimination.

CASE STUDY (6)

The interviews for the new practice manager finished at 1.00 p.m. and the partners were astonished at how tired they were. It was clear that if there was a disagreement it was going to be difficult to get two of the partners to stay for a full discussion. Tom and Bill would have preferred waiting until Monday as they were anxious to rejoin their families. However, when they each summarized the candidates it was clear there were two front runners: the accountant Cathy Colby, and Simon Hayes from the Family Health Services Authority (FHSA). Unfortunately, because they had not organized their interviewing in a systematic way, there were gaps in both the candidates' CVs which were worrying. Veronica offered to ring them up and get the information in time to decide at the next partners' meeting on Monday. Bill was very enthusiastic about that idea and in the end they agreed that both should be called back for a second interview, if possible that Monday evening.

Veronica reported back on Monday morning that both were prepared to come back, though both were slightly irritated by the process, mainly because they had not been warned in advance. On Monday afternoon Simon rang to say that he had thought the matter over and had discussed it with his manager. He felt that the selection process confirmed that general practice did not offer the managerial professionalism that he sought. As he had been offered enhanced job opportunities with the FHSA, he felt that he should stay where he was, and withdrew his application. The partners were very deflated.

Cathy arrived in the evening and was seen by them all, and they were all impressed. They felt happy and agreed they would offer her the post then and there. To their horror Cathy was not bowled over by the offer. 'Perhaps I could think about it for a day or two' she said. 'There are a number of things I need to consider.' Bill hastened to say that they would be happy to give her time to think about what was obviously a major career move and asked if there was anything else they could tell her. They all reassured her that they were anxious to have her on board as their professional manager. She then asked about pension arrangements, which confused them, and her questions about maternity leave and sick pay – which they had not sorted out properly – left them wondering if they had offered the job to someone who was going to have six children immediately, and go down with a debilitating if not fatal illness! They had not thought about making the offer conditional upon their getting references or a medical opinion as to her suitability for the post.

Cathy laughed at the end of the discussion and said she would have to take the job as they so obviously needed someone to sort them out! And she supposed she would have to write her own contract!

'What contract?' asked Bill.

Post-interview procedures

The unsuccessful candidates

Once the successful candidate has accepted the offer it is important to write to all those who were unsuccessful. Some may telephone to ask why they had not got the job. There is no legal obligation to respond but it is helpful for candidates to be aware of the reasons. They have, after all, invested time in the organization. Any response should not address the personality of the candidate but concentrate on the areas of experience, qualifications and so on which the interview panel felt were strongest in the successful candidate.

Medical examinations

Ironically, many general practitioners are reluctant to ask questions or probe applicants about their health. Unless the position is extraordinarily demanding the completion of a health questionnaire, followed if necessary by a medical examination, is sufficient for most positions in general practice. It is important, however, to ensure physical and mental fitness for the post.

When it is necessary for medical records to be obtained from another medical practitioner, the requirements of the Access to Medical Reports Act 1988 must be observed, with consent to the application for information being obtained from the individual concerned. It is advisable for the practice to pay the cost of the medical examination and any related travelling expenses.

The issue of staff as patients needs also to be addressed by any practice where there are alternative options nearby. Chapter 6 (on performance appraisal) and Chapter 7 (on discipline) make clear the difficulties that may arise if the employer relationship is confused with the employee/doctor/patient relationship.

Documentation

The recruitment process must be properly documented. Accurate records of interviews and the reasons for selection and rejection at each stage should be maintained. This is in accordance with the ACAS Codes of Practice referred to earlier (see page 23). It is very important that all organizations follow these codes. The codes themselves do not impose any legal obligations. However, if their recommendations are not observed, breaches of the law may result. The codes' provisions are admissible in evidence before an industrial tribunal and if any provision appears to the tribunal to be relevant to the proceedings it must be taken into account.

The next chapter addresses the area that puzzled Bill String, that is the contractual relationship which exists between the employer and employee as soon as the offer of employment is accepted.

2 How to Employ Staff

THE relationship between employer and employee is a legal one, embodied in the contract of employment. The contract is at the heart of the complex employment legislation in this country. Employers and managers have to be aware of the nature of that contract and their legal rights and responsibilities. Appendix B lists the major legislation involved.

The legal requirements

Like any other employers, general practitioners are bound by law in their employment of staff and have to grapple with its effects when hiring, reorganizing or dismissing staff. There is considerable evidence of general practitioners neglecting staff matters, and until recently a sizeable majority of practice staff did not have written contracts (Ellis, 1990). Since the Contracts of Employment Act 1963 – now replaced by the Employment Protection Consolidation Act (EPCA) 1978 – all employers have been required to give written statements of the main terms and conditions of employment to their staff. Since April 1990 (Secretaries of State for Health 1990), much attention has been given to the subject largely as a result of FHSAs requiring copies of written statements for new staff, and for those staff whose terms and conditions practices wish to alter.

It is important to understand and differentiate between the contract, the written contract and the written statement of principal terms.

Contract

If one person employs another, then there is a 'contract' between them even if nothing is in writing. There will always be certain areas of such a contract which cannot be codified but which nevertheless form an integral part of the total contract. There are many understandings between employer and employee which reflect goodwill and 'give and take' which cannot and should not be documented.

However the advantages of a verbal contract – informality and simplicity – are heavily outweighed by the disadvantages – imprecision, unreliability, vulnerability to misinterpretation and difficulty in enforcing or changing the terms.

Written contract

It is useful, indeed highly desirable in any event, that the main terms of the contract are put in writing. The phrase 'written contract' usually means the document or documents which contain these terms. At one end of the scale this could be the lengthy and comprehensive 'contract of service' prepared by solicitors and signed by both parties, or possibly a letter from the employer offering the job and setting out the main terms.

Written statement of principal terms

Although the employment contract does not have to be in writing to be valid and enforceable, it is a legal requirement that every employee should be given a 'written statement of particulars of certain terms'. This may be a printed sheet or a letter, or the full written contract itself may embody and include these 'principal terms'.

Although the law requires this written statement to be given within 13 weeks*, there is no actual penalty or fine if the employer does not provide the written statement. However, employers ignore the requirements at their peril, as the sanctions for not giving the written statement are:

1 Employees can apply to the industrial tribunal for terms to be clarified and for the statement to be prepared; if there are any terms which are in doubt, then the tribunal is likely to give the benefit of the doubt to the employee.
2 If the employer is unfortunate enough to be involved in any tribunal proceedings (eg for unfair dismissal), the first question from the

---

* At the time of writing this requirement is being amended under the new Trade Union Reform and Employment Rights Bill. If the proposals in the bill are passed as law, employers will be required to provide a written statement within two months of commencing service to all staff who work eight hours a week or more.

tribunal chairman is likely to be a request to see the contract or written particulars, and an embarrassed explanation as to why this does not exist is likely to give a bad or prejudicial impression of the employer from the start.

All employees of the practice are entitled to receive a written contract in accordance with EPCA 1978. However, employee status is not always clear cut in general practice. Attached staff, self-employed or agency people are not employed by the practice and should not therefore receive a written contract of employment. If there are staff in the practice whose status is ambiguous, a solicitor should be consulted before issuing a written contract. Examples of standard written employment contracts can be obtained from the British Medical Association (BMA) and AHCPA. Their addresses can be found in Appendix C.

What is a contract?*

A contract is an agreement between two or more parties which is enforceable in law. The elements of an employment contract are:

- expressed terms including 'incorporated terms'
- implied terms, which can be either generally implied, or custom and practice
- statutory overlay.

Express terms

The express terms of a contract are those which most people think of as 'the contract of employment'. These are terms which have been spelled out in so many words, whether in writing or under a verbal agreement. Certain of these express terms must be put in writing and given to the employee within 13 weeks (*see above) of commencing employment. These are set out in Box 2.1.

* At the time of writing the Trade Union Reform and Employment Rights Bill is in Committee stage of its passage through Parliament. If the proposals in the bill are adopted and passed as law then the requirements for written contracts of employment will be affected.

Box 2.1: Legal requirements for individual information

- The parties to the contract, ie the employer's name and the employee's name.
- Date the employment began.
- Continuity of employment, ie whether or not employment with another employer (eg another practice) will count as continuous employment. This is particularly significant as the majority of legal rights employees enjoy are determined by length of service.
- Title of the job.
- Scale or rate of remuneration, or method of calculating remuneration.
- Intervals at which salary/wages are paid (monthly, weekly, etc).
- Hours of working including rota details and Bank Holiday arrangements.
- Any terms and conditions relating to:
  - holiday entitlement and holiday pay
  - sick leave and sick pay
  - whether or not there is any pension scheme other than the State scheme with details (if appropriate)
  - length of notice which the employee is obliged to give and entitled to receive to terminate the contract. After four weeks of continuous service employees are entitled by law to receive notice of one week, and in addition one week's notice for each completed year of continuous service up to 12 weeks' notice. Thus:

Length of service	Notice entitlement
from 1 month up to 2 years	1 week
2 years	2 weeks
3 years	3 weeks
12 years	12 weeks

Fifteen years' service would attract a legal entitlement to 12 weeks' notice. Employers can of course offer more generous notice periods. What they cannot do is 'contract out' of these minimum periods by stipulating less than the minimum.

There are also a number of items which might not be thought of as part of the 'day-to-day' terms but which are required to be given to the employee, and these are listed in Box 2.2.

Box 2.2: Other information which employees are legally entitled to receive
- Any disciplinary rules or reference to a document accessible to the employee which specifies such rules.
- The person to whom the employee can appeal if he/she is dissatisfied with any disciplinary decision relating to him/her.
- The person to whom the employee should address any grievances and the manner in which this should be done.
- Whether or not a contracting-out certificate for State Earnings Related Pension Scheme (SERPS) is in force.

In the written contract, the employer can include other 'express terms' over and above those which are mentioned above, eg:

- standards of dress required
- that an employee can be called upon to undertake suitable alternative work to fit in with the needs of the practice
- redundancy policy
- the normal retirement age
- specific obligations where an employee is required to drive a car in the course of their duty.

'Incorporated terms' refer to the express incorporation of terms determined by national and/or local collective agreements. For instance, many practice employment contracts will contain statements that rates of pay are to be determined by the Whitley Council (*see* Appendix C). This is an incorporated term.

Implied terms

There are many rights and obligations on either side which are left unexpressed and unspecified. The general rule is that a term will be implied in a contract if it is necessary to give it business efficacy or if it is so obvious that it does not need expressing. It is common, particularly where disagreements arise between employers and employees, to focus on the written and expressed terms of the contract at the expense of the implied terms.

Those implied terms present in *all* employment contracts are specified in Box 2.3.

Box 2.3: Implied terms
- Employee's duties: fidelity
    obedience
    to work with diligence and care
- Employer's duties: to act reasonably
    to maintain a relationship of trust and
    confidence with the employee
    to provide a safe system of work and a
    safe working environment
    to provide wages (there is no general duty
    to provide work)
- Custom and practice

Employee's duties

Fidelity – to serve the employer

The relationship between an employer and employee is a personal one. The duty to serve means to serve in accordance with the terms of the contract. For instance, it is not a breach of contract to be absent from work as long as the absence is catered for in the contract – eg holiday and sickness absence. Absences outside the contract need to be authorized by the employer if they are not to be viewed as a breach of contract as a result of which, in theory, the employer is able to claim damages for breach of contract or, more usually, to discipline the employee and in extreme cases, to dismiss the employee. Any such dismissal must be within the legislation relating to unfair dismissal and at all times the employer must act reasonably.

Example 2.1
Sheila, a receptionist, failed to report for work on a Monday morning. The following day she returned to work and claimed that her absence was due to illness. Her contract required her to contact her employer on the first day of absence, and consequently she was in breach of her contract of employment. However, as this was not a common occurrence and she was

a good and diligent employee in all other respects, the practice manager merely drew her attention to the terms of the contract and pointed out the reason behind the rule, namely to ensure the practice could make proper provision for covering her absence.

Obedience

The obligation of obedience does not mean that the employee must do anything the employer asks of them. Employees are required to obey only lawful instructions within the scope of the contract.

Example 2.2
A practice manager requested a receptionist to undertake cleaning duties when the practice cleaner went on holiday. The receptionist declined on the grounds that it was neither in her job title nor in her job description. Although the practice manager argued and was very angry with the receptionist for not obeying her, she knew that, while not asking anything unlawful of her staff, she was asking her to do something outside the terms of the receptionist's contract.

Competence and duty of care

Except where specific training needs are agreed, employees accept job offers on the understanding that they are capable of doing the job for which they have been employed. As this is difficult to authenticate at interview, most contracts contain a probationary period which allows the employer the opportunity to assess the employee's competence. The successful completion of the probationary period does not prevent the employer from later addressing issues of incompetence and negligence through the disciplinary procedure. The implied duty of competence and care remains a term of the contract until the contract is terminated.

Duty of good faith

If the employment contract is to operate, there must be trust and confidence between both parties. The degree of this will often be determined by the status of the employee. Higher standards of good faith would be demanded for an accountant, for example, than for an unskilled labourer. In many jobs (and this is true for posts within general practice where surgeries demand a high level of confidentiality) it is advisable to specify as an express term that an employee has a duty of confidentiality which continues after they have left the practice's employment. Clearly this has disciplinary connotations, and these are dealt with in Chapter 7 and the case study (14).

Employer's duties

Acting reasonably

The overriding duty of all employers is to act reasonably and not to destroy the relationship of trust and confidence between the parties. This pervades the contractual relationship, and industrial tribunals take it very seriously. There can never be a hard-and-fast legal definition as to what is reasonable behaviour and each case is determined on its merits. The standard to be applied seems to be very variable and is often influenced by the size of the organization. Reasonable behaviour by a large multinational in finding alternative work for employees under notice of redundancy may be very different from reasonable behaviour expected of a small practice with fewer resources.

Personal behaviour between employer and employee is also subject to the test of reasonableness. Comments to employees which destroy the mutual confidence between the parties can be viewed by industrial tribunals as constructive dismissal. In the case of Courtaulds Northern Textiles v Andrew 1979 (IRLR 1984), the supervisor in the course of a row shouted at an employee 'Well, you can't do the bloody job anyway'. The employee resigned, claiming constructive dismissal. The Employment Appeal Tribunal ruled that unfair dismissal had occurred because the comment gratuitously destroyed the mutual confidence between the parties. The management in the form of the supervisor did not really believe that the employee could not do the job.

Any criticisms of an employee's behaviour or performance must be dealt with within the terms of the contract – through informal counselling or via the disciplinary procedure – and should not be undertaken in a manner or place likely to humiliate the employee. Shouting at a receptionist in the middle of the waiting area is not reasonable behaviour.

Example 2.3

One of the partners in a practice discovered that for the third time that week one of the receptionists had given her the wrong medical notes for a patient. This was only discovered when the patient was in the consulting room. Understandably embarrassed and very annoyed, the doctor left the consulting room and delivered a heated rebuke to the receptionist concerned in reception in full view of the waiting patients and other staff.

The doctor vented her anger and felt better. The receptionist, however, was extremely distressed and felt humiliated. She told her solicitor husband who wrote to the doctor concerned, pointing out that she was in breach of the implied terms of her contract with the receptionist to act reasonably. The doctor's criticism of the receptionist should have been delivered in private. The doctor was mortified and frightened of the possible consequences, as were her partners. They persuaded her to give a sincere and graceful apology for the manner of her rebuke to the receptionist in public, which the receptionist accepted. The problem of the incorrect notes was then addressed calmly.

Health and safety

The detailed regulations of the duties of the employer in relation to health and safety are set out in the Health and Safety at Work Act 1974. In addition there are implied terms, as set out in Box 2.4.

Box 2.4: Health and Safety implied terms
- To select reasonably competent employees.
- To provide adequate materials.
- To provide a safe system of working.

To provide wages

The express terms of the contract will specify the amount of wages and the method and frequency of payment. If for some reason there is no express term (very rare these days), then the implied term of the contract is held by the courts to be that the employer will provide wages for the work undertaken.

Failure to pay the agreed salary is breach of contract and the employee may sue for damages in the civil court and/or resign and claim constructive dismissal. However, the duty to pay wages is contingent upon the employee performing his or her side of the bargain. If an employee refuses to work or goes on strike, the general principle of 'no work, no pay' applies.

To provide work

This is an ambiguous area of the law. Where the provision of work determines the amount an employee is paid – piece work, payment by results and so on – the implied term of the contract is that the employer is bound to provide work in order for the employee to earn a living. Many contracts specify circumstances under which the employer has the right not to provide work, eg suspension from work on full pay during a disciplinary investigation (see Chapter 7).

Miscellaneous

There are other implied terms. For example in Roberts v Toyota (GB) Ltd (1981 EATO 614/80), the area sales manager's contract expressly provided that he would have a company car for use on company business. The implied term was that he should hold a valid driving licence; the express term would be virtually meaningless without it. This case was brought to an industrial tribunal when the area manager claimed unsuccessfully that he had been unfairly dismissed when he lost his driving licence. This could apply if a practice with branch surgeries required certain staff to be able to use the practice car to travel between branch surgeries, if no other means of transport was available.

Custom and practice

Other specific terms may be implied in employment contracts if they are regularly adopted in a particular trade or industry or in a particular locality or in a particular practice. Customs and practices are often quite quickly established in organizations and it is wise to be aware that where a particular custom is introduced it may, once firmly established, become part of the contract of employment.

Example 2.4

A practice over a number of years gave Christmas bonuses to all the staff. They decided one year that the practice income was too reduced to enable them to do so. Instead of getting the staff's consent, they simply did not give the bonuses. They found themselves arguing about a change in contract which had not been negotiated, even though it was 'only' based on custom and practice. It was clear that if they had shared the practice aims and performance with the staff, the staff themselves might have suggested an all-round 'tightening of the belt', including of course demonstrably reduced drawings by the doctors themselves.

Statutory overlay

Statutory terms cover the legal provisions relating to employment relationships. The contract of employment will only override these if it exceeds statutory minimum employment rights of the employee. Consequently, as new employment legislation is introduced, so the contract of employment is changed irrespective of whether the employer reviews it or not.

Example 2.5

A practice receptionist became pregnant and was informed by the practice manager that she could have only 20 weeks' maternity leave after the baby was born because the practice was running into holiday periods for the rest of the staff. Her contract was an informal list of terms, of which one covered maternity leave, and stated that it would be subject to the exigencies of the practice. In fact, as she had been employed at the practice for over two years, she was legally entitled to receive 29 weeks' maternity leave after the birth of the baby. The practice had to provide proper maternity cover to ensure they complied with the law, regardless of the fact that the written contract had been accepted by the receptionist.

For clarity the principal minimum statutory individual employment rights relevant to practice staff are detailed in Appendix D, but there are some that need discussion as they will reflect and document the style and nature of the employee/employer relationship each practice will want to introduce. With very limited exceptions, an employer and an employee are not allowed to contract out of the terms implied by employment legislation.

Drafting the contract

Drafting the contract is a major opportunity for a practice to review its current employment policies. Documenting such terms and conditions is not only helpful for staff and the practice but also provides a source of material when promoting the practice through job and recruitment advertisements (*see* Chapter 1).

Some areas which may warrant consideration for inclusion in drafting a contract may include the following.

1 *Holiday leave*. The practice may wish to reward long-serving staff by attaching holiday leave increases to length of service. It may also want to make provision for special leave, eg for bereavement, public and civil duties or study. It will certainly need to have a policy for deciding who gets priority if holidays coincide with those of other staff.

2 *Sickness*. One of the most common areas of dispute in practices concerns sick leave and pay. Disputes arise particularly if staff are not clear as to when and who they should inform when they are ill, or when self and medical certificates should be submitted. Practices will find it helpful to have clear rules to limit the chances of misunderstanding. Furthermore, they may wish to have a policy for handling staff who appear to have excessive sick leave.

3 *Pension and pension schemes*. Even if the practice has no occupa-

tional pension scheme, specifying retirement ages is advisable. Some staff may have commenced employment many years ago and will not have received any communication as to their retirement age. It may seem obvious what it is – 60 for women, 65 for men – but it is not uncommon for people to work beyond these ages. The current state pension ages for men and women in the United Kingdom are being reviewed by EEC law. Indeed some employers have been taken to the European Court for discrimination between the sexes on this very issue (Barber v Guardian Royal Exchange). On 7 November 1987 an amendment to the Sex Discrimination Act 1986 came into effect which made unlawful discrimination between the sexes through any provision relating to retirement which concerned promotion, transfer, training, dismissal or demotion. The most significant effect of this amendment is that employers may no longer offer different retirement ages to men and women in comparable positions in the same organization.

4 *Flexibility*. Contracts of employment are not static. Circumstances change and events occur which impinge on the employer/staff relationship. If any of these can be anticipated then it is wise to make provision for them in the written contract.

Example 2.6
A practice planned to develop a branch surgery in two years' time. It was clear that main surgery staff might on occasion be required to work in the branch surgery. New written terms of service were drawn up to include this requirement in the contract of employment for new staff, but also with existing staff, by agreement.

---

5 *Health and safety, and equal opportunities*. Although there is no legal requirement to include reference to either of these two areas in the written contract, employers are legally required to produce a health and safety policy and to abide by the Health and Safety at Work Act 1974 and the Sex and Race Discrimination Acts of 1975 and 1976. A practice may wish to express its commitment to both these areas by way of developing policies that can be included in the written contract.

6 *Disciplinary procedures*. These are addressed in Chapter 6.

During the process of contract design it is important to discuss and agree terms with the existing staff. Producing a *fait accompli* will not help if staff are opposed to any of the terms and conditions. Genuine consultation is not only good management practice but advisable particularly if, through the production of the written contract, the practice is introducing new or changing current terms and conditions of employment (*see* Example 2.6).

Although the written contract is a legal document it should be in plain English. Using legal jargon does not in any way increase the contract's legal standing but it does detrimentally affect its efficacy. A contract peppered with legal jargon will also convey the impression that the practice views its staff in a very formal way. Clearly, in most practices, relationships are characterized by informality and mutual dependency. The contract therefore should be clearly written and in a style which reflects and promotes the style and culture of the practice. It is worthwhile for a practice to find a solicitor who can achieve this.

Finally, the written contract should be given to staff and, although there is no legal obligation for the contract to be signed, it is advisable for both parties to do so.

Providing a signed written contract for each member of staff containing the comprehensive details of the terms and conditions of employment may seem rather cumbersome. The most popular format overcomes this obstacle by producing a one- or two-page contract that contains the terms peculiar to each employee:

- employee's name
- date employment began (and continuity of employment)
- job title
- salary
- hours of work

and merely refers to other documents (larger practices may have a staff handbook, for instance) where further details can be found.

The offer of employment

The actual contract of employment between the employer and the employee begins as soon as the successful candidate accepts the offer of employment – *see* case study (6). Promises made at interview which are false or are later withdrawn can constitute breach of contract, particularly if put in the offer of employment. If such promises have a financial element, for example an increase in salary within a certain period, then the employee can claim damages in a civil court. It is important, therefore, that offers of employment are scrutinized to ensure that restrictions or qualifications to promises made are included in writing in the offer of employment. Box 2.5 gives some examples.

Box 2.5: Restrictions and qualifications to employment offers
Restrictions:
* 'subject to satisfactory references'
* 'subject to the satisfactory outcome of any medical examination'

Qualifications:
* use the term 'established' job rather than 'permanent' job to avoid any implication of a job for life
* use the phrase 'after the successful completion of a probationary period of . . . . . . months your employment will be confirmed'
* qualify any training needs identified at the interview by the words 'according to the needs and resources of the practice'.

Changing the contract

Many employers wrongly assume that a contract of employment cannot be changed after it has been agreed. This view is often expressed to excuse or justify not issuing written contracts of employment. In fact most contracts change at least annually as a result of salary increases, without either party formally giving notice or formally accepting such changes. Changes which are of benefit to employees – salary rises, increased holidays and so on – can be safely introduced without fear of the employee seeking recourse at an industrial tribunal or a civil court. It is those changes which are of no benefit or perceived benefit to employees which must be handled with skill and sensitivity, and within the law.

The law requires that any change to the main terms and conditions of employment (as listed in Box 2.1) should be notified to the employee within one month of the change being implemented. However, employers need to do far more than this if they are to avoid civil court action for breach of contract and industrial tribunals for claims of unfair dismissal.

Employer's remedies and practices

If there is, or there may be opposition to a proposed change, and the practice nevertheless decides to press ahead, it is important that a few golden rules are followed in order to avoid or limit the damages.

First, all staff who are likely to be affected by the proposal need to be informed of the reason for the change and the process which will be used in introducing and implementing such change (Plant, 1987). This should be done as follows.

- Everyone affected is informed, preferably in writing, of the proposed change.
- The reasons are 'reasonable', clear and in the interests of the practice.
- Staff are consulted and where possible, objections accommodated.
- Each employee is offered, in writing, the change to their contract.

If at this stage the offer is agreed, the second step is to gain acceptance in writing and implement. However, if some staff will not agree, then the partners need to make a decision whether or not to implement the variation. If the change is necessary to the success and functioning of the practice, it may be judicious at this stage to seek legal advice. Any legal advice sought should address the following options and courses of action open to the practice if it decides to go ahead.

- Staff who continue to resist the change should be clearly warned that the only other option will be to terminate their *existing contracts*.
- If at this stage, and after continuing to consult, some staff steadfastly refuse to accept the change, notice should now be given to them in writing, that their *existing contracts* will be terminated. The notice period should be at least the statutory minimum (*see* Box 2.1) or the notice specified in their written contracts, whichever is the longer.

- This letter should end with an offer of re-engagement at the end of the notice period on the new terms.

Giving notice merely to change the contract will be viewed as imposing the change without agreement. It is vital, therefore, that the employees are put under notice to terminate their existing contracts. Staff who refuse the new offer, and whose contracts are therefore terminated, may still bring a claim for unfair dismissal. Demonstrating sound reasons for the change and a comprehensive consultative exercise will probably result in the dismissal being found fair at an industrial tribunal.

There is a second option in managing those staff who simply refuse to accept the change where such a refusal involves non-co-operation – for example where an employee simply refuses to receive training in order to operate a computer. The practice can dismiss for disobedience or non-co-operation. The practice's disciplinary procedure needs to be used in disciplining the member of staff (*see* Chapter 7). An industrial tribunal will probably view such a course of action less sympathetically than the process of terminating existing contracts and offering new ones. However, if the practice has acted reasonably and particularly if it is an isolated employee who is refusing to accept the change, then the practice may be adjudged to have dismissed fairly. For instance, in the case of Cresswell v Board of Inland Revenue (1984 ICR508), it was held that an employee is expected to adapt to new methods and techniques of working provided that the employer arranges for them to receive the necessary training in the new skills, and that the nature of the work does not alter so radically that it is outside the contractual obligations of the employee.

Imposed change

There are two remedies which an employee can seek if a change is imposed on their contract of employment. First, if the change has resulted in a financial loss to the employee, the employee can sue for damages in a civil court. Unlike industrial tribunals, civil courts will not consider the reasonableness of the change. An assessment of the financial loss will be made and the employer ordered to pay damages. Employees do not have to resign to bring a civil court action. They can, if they wish, continue working under protest whilst the case is being considered. Clearly any change which did not financially penalize the employee would not attract damages.

Example 2.7
A practice, which has previously awarded annual increments to all staff, decided to alter this process to a system where increments were awarded on the level of performance reached over the previous year. Those staff who had not performed to the standard required were not awarded an increment. The practice toyed with the idea of imposing this change, but when they suggested it to the practice manager she warned that one or two of the staff planned their expenditure for the forthcoming year on the basis of receiving a regular increment. It was possible that they would think it worth their while to pursue the practice in the courts. She told them that employees could sue in a civil court for damages, both in this case and if there were any alteration to the terms and conditions of employment which impacted on salaries to the employees' disadvantage.

Secondly, even those changes which do not attract a financial disadvantage to the employee may cause a member of staff to seek redress through an industrial tribunal. Any fundamental breach of contract may result in the employee resigning and claiming constructive unfair dismissal in an industrial tribunal.

Example 2.8
A practice had undergone many changes over the previous two years. These developments caused the partners to review the capability of their practice manager who had held the post for many years. It was decided to appoint a better qualified practice manager and to designate the current post holder as deputy practice manager. The practice did not reduce the current manager's salary or any of her entitlements. She suffered no financial loss. The change was announced and imposed. There was no consultation.

The practice manager resigned and lodged a claim at an industrial tribunal for constructive dismissal. Her claim was based on three instances of breach of contract.

1 One of the express and statutory terms of her written contract was her job title, which had been changed, resulting in loss of status.

2 One of the implied terms of her contract was that her employer acted reasonably. This had been breached because she had not been consulted, and she had lost status and felt humiliated.

3 The implied terms – of maintaining a relationship of trust and confidence – had also been breached. Having never received any indication that her performance was not meeting the needs of the practice, the practice manager now felt that she could no longer trust the integrity of the partners. Her confidence in them as employers had been fundamentally breached.

The advice to the practice was that this claim would probably succeed at tribunal. The change was fundamental and therefore caused the employee to resign. The employee acted quickly, as she knew that any delay in voicing objections and resigning would damage her claim. The industrial tribunal would consider the reasonableness of the employer's position and their attempt to show that there were good reasons for the change and whether the manner and method of introducing the change was reasonable. The practice's solicitor advised the partners to settle before the tribunal hearing.

Although the above examples describe legal avenues for redress, the employee has a third option, depending on the nature of the change: simply to refuse the change.

Example 2.9
A practice decided to alter its surgery hours in response to the results of a recent comprehensive patient survey. The alteration necessitated a change to the hours of work of four part-time staff. The number of hours worked each week were not altered only when those hours were worked. This decision was announced, without consultation, and two of the affected staff continued reporting for work as before. Although the

written element of their contracts of employment did not specify when their hours of work were to be undertaken, the fact that for an established period of time they had reported for and left work at specific times on specific days of the week meant that the practice was in breach of their contracts of employment.

The above examples are instances where changes have been imposed, to the detriment of employees, without consultation. Change is possible and is increasingly necessary in general practice, a profession which is undergoing major changes and innovations, many of which will impinge on employment contracts. So how can practices change contracts of employment?

Gaining consent

The first step to take is to gain acceptance of the change. It is not only prudent but also good management practice genuinely to consult staff and persuade them through well thought-out proposals and clear reasoning. Such consultation should be done directly and not delegated to other staff. Second-hand explanations, particularly by someone who may be opposed to change, will seriously damage the case. The change cannot be contractually binding if the employee does not consent to it. It is therefore important to consider any objections and if the practice's needs can still be met, to be prepared to compromise.

Example 2.10
The needs of the practice in Example 2.8 could have been met quite differently as shown in another health centre where the practice manager was told of the partners' thoughts on the new areas of work and associated skills the practice now wanted. She was consulted fully so that she understood the reasons why the practice needed these skills. They were demonstrated to her as reasonable and directly related to the developments within the practice. The practice manager was then given time to consider the proposed change – in this instance to appoint a new manager. Her objections and suggestions were given real

consideration, and, where possible, accommodated. In the
event, she decided that she did not have the relevant skills or
expertise, and opted to take redundancy terms (*see* Chapter 9).

After gaining agreement, acceptance must be positive, unequivocal and
unconditional for the change to be legally binding. Such agreement
need not be in writing; it can be by conduct. As with issuing the
written employment contract, it is better to gain written acceptance.
Disputes hinging on 'your word against mine' can then be avoided.
Receiving no response cannot be interpreted as acceptance, nor can
making the change and insisting that it has become legally binding
because the employee has not rejected it. If changes are introduced
and employees work under the new terms without voicing any objections then it is safe to assume that the change has been accepted.
However, nothing can replace wide and genuine consultation as the
most effective and safe method of introducing change.

The acceptance must be unconditional; staff cannot accept some
parts of an offer and reject others where it constitutes a package. An
offer of an increase in salary tied to an increase in responsibility, for
example, has to be accepted or rejected in its totality. The higher
salary cannot be accepted if the responsibility is rejected.

Consulting and gaining acceptance is an integral part of the
employer's duty to act reasonably. Acting reasonably involves both
the way the change has been introduced and the change itself – is it
reasonable in the particular circumstances of the practice?

Of course, many practices will issue contracts which allow for
change. It makes sense to ensure that the written contract is drafted
to give a balance between certainty and flexibility. The contract should
cater for the evolving needs of the practice so that terms and conditions
can be altered whilst remaining within the contractual obligation
which binds them. But it is important to ensure that such clauses are
reasonable to the employee. Civil courts and tribunals are extremely
reluctant to ratify a *carte blanche* clause to rewrite the contact unilat-
erally. Even where there is a clause specifying the right to change –
for example introducing weekend work – practices are still obliged to
give reasonable notice of any change.

Preventing determined staff who wish to bring a case of either civil
action for breach of contract and/or an unfair dismissal claim to an
industrial tribunal is not easy. However, by handling contract changes

legally and skilfully, and by embarking on a genuine consultation exercise, the damages suffered can be limited.

It is important to understand that the contract of employment is a two-party legal document. Just as employees are expected to work with diligence, care, fidelity and obedience (and the disciplinary procedure is there to deal with breaches of these implied terms – *see* Chapter 7), so too are employers expected to act reasonably and maintain good working relationships with staff. It is a contractual obligation.

A well constructed and carefully drafted written contract will promote good relations within the practice and foster the smooth introduction of changes and variations to the orginally agreed terms and conditions of employment. A good introduction to the practice through a well thought-out and comprehensive induction programme will also promote a sound basis for the relationship. This is the subject of the next chapter.

3 How to Introduce and Induct New Staff

IT is all too easy to breathe a sigh of relief once the new recruit has accepted the offer of employment and the written contract has been issued. The temptation is to see the new employee as an immediate asset who will contribute effectively to the work of the practice from day one. Yet the recruitment process is in fact not completed until the successful candidate has been thoroughly inducted. A poorly managed induction can sabotage an effective recruitment process.

The purpose of induction

The purposes of induction are summarized in Box 3.1. The basic objective is to help the new recruit settle down to the new job as soon as possible. It is as relevant for trainees and new partners as for new members of staff, so for the purposes of this chapter the word 'employee' includes all new people who will be working in the practice.

Box 3.1 The purposes of induction
- To help obtain the best possible performance from the new employee in the shortest possible time.
- To help retain the services of the employee.
- To give the employee an understanding and appreciation of the practice, provide the context within which their job operates, an understanding of the main terms and conditions of employment and an awareness of the roles of the other team members.

What is induction?

Starting a new job is a particularly anxious time for new staff. Even the most self-confident people, regardless of the status of the post to which they have been appointed, suffer some apprehension before and during the first few months of working for a new employer. If this anxiety is not managed by the practice it can interfere with the employee's capacity to learn (and *all* new jobs entail a learning element), and in extreme cases can prompt the person to resign. Preparing a formal and informal induction programme helps to allay anxieties and ensures that the new colleague contributes to the practice early on in their service.

Empathy with new colleagues does not come naturally. Tasks which existing employees and managers find easy will be new and may be even frightening to the new employee. For example, the independent contractor status of general practitioners is a highly complex concept which will not be known to new reception staff. Equally the National Health Service (NHS) is a giant of an organization but a general practice is normally quite small. Disappointment may be felt by employees when they realize, after their appointment, that there is no larger organization offering promotional opportunities unless they were to leave the practice. Such disappointment can be modified through a good induction programme.

There are no set rules. The content, method, time period and the person to do the inducting will be determined by the structure of the practice and the responsibilities of the job. It is normal for the employee's direct manager – a partner for the practice manager, senior receptionist for the receptionist – to undertake the induction process.

The basic needs of all new employees are set out in Box 3.2.

Box 3.2: Basic induction needs
All new recruits need to become familiar with:
- the people
- the surroundings
- the job
- the terms and conditions of employment
- health and safety
- the management style and structure
- the organization

CASE STUDY (7)

Cathy Colby started on 1 March as practice manager at the John Street Health Centre. Her strengths lay in the financial and staff management side of the job – clearly her knowledge of general practice and indeed the Health Service more generally was limited. Unfortunately the partners did not recognize this. It was Cathy herself who had to ask for their ideas on suitable reading so that she could gain some background, but their response was merely to suggest the weekly general practice magazines. They did not attempt to see or contact her between the interview and the negotiated starting date. Indeed when she suggested that she should meet the staff prior to taking up the post, the partners agreed that it would be a good idea, but did not arrange a date or tell the staff that this had been suggested. They all believed it would become clear when she arrived and they could explain it all then. They felt that she would pick up the management and administration of the practice quickly because 'it is largely common sense, isn't it?' They did not recognize the importance for Cathy to understand the key issues facing general practice, or the political and clinical context in which they would expect her to operate.

As a consequence Cathy felt she made two blunders early on – the first was in trying to change the treatment room appointment times to relieve pressure on the reception desk, without understanding fully the inter-professional rivalries involved, and without talking it through with the partnership. She had to withdraw her proposal in the face of angry staff and received no support or understanding from her employers. She accepted her error, and made friends with the staff, but did not feel the partners took their share of the blame. They should have made sure she understood that there was a sensitivity over the nurse/doctor relationship generally, and the current policies within the practice vis à vis the nurse/manager roles.

Her second 'mistake' was to make an appointment with the practice account-ant to talk through the accounts, again without talking to the partners. They had not told the accountant that they had a new practice manager who was financially trained. As a consequence he resisted her questioning and refused to discuss with her matters that he had only discussed with partners hitherto. Cathy came back from the appointment feeling humiliated, very upset and angry.

She felt both situations were directly due to lack of guidance, direction and induction by the partners. In addition she discovered that the partners had been very secretive with the staff about her appointment, as a result of which the staff were anxious and a little hostile, and certainly did not help her get things right. Cathy asked to see the middle partner, Veronica Irons, with whom she felt most empathy, and said that she was most unhappy at the lack of induction. She was thinking of resigning, as she was beginning to feel that this was not the right post for her, nor she the right person for the practice.

The components of induction

The people

A new place of work is bewildering and being introduced to 15 people on the first morning may not be helpful. New colleagues need to be introduced first to those with whom they will be working closest, and gradually introduced to the rest of the practice team as the need and occasion arises. A formal introduction to each partner will emphasize the team nature of the practice, particularly if each partner is responsible for a particular activity within the practice – finance, staff, clinical protocols, education and so on. It may also be helpful to allocate a mentor to ease the new person into the organization, charging an experienced, friendly member of staff with the duty of looking after the new recruit during their first week or so at the practice. Such a mentor can provide the information and advice the new recruit will seek from time to time. However this informal induction process should not replace the formal training and coaching all new people require.

The surroundings

A tour of the premises and the location of the staff room, the toilets, washrooms, first-aid box and so on are the parts of the induction of new staff which should be undertaken within the first day.

The job

Before the employee has started, some form of training programme needs to have been thought out and written down. If the recruitment and selection procedure has been effective, there will already be a list of areas where the new employee requires immediate and longer-term training and development. In addition to this list, each major task of the job needs to be analysed in terms of the information, skills, training and experience the new person will need in order to achieve a satisfactory level of competence. Involving the new person in the implementation of the job induction programme will help allay anxieties and emphasize the importance with which the practice views quality work and the value and worth of employees to the practice.

This may sound long-winded and time-consuming. However, where there is more than one post for positions common in the practice –

such as receptionists – this training programme can be adapted and used repeatedly whenever a new receptionist starts work. The consequences of a patient's complaint being badly handled by an untrained receptionist will put this induction commitment, and the time spent on it, into perspective!

The induction gives the opportunity to set the standards of performance and conduct the practice expects of its staff. If this period is neglected, new staff may pick up bad habits and indifferent attitudes from some existing long-serving staff. 'Getting it right' at the beginning is much easier than having to rectify unhelpful attitudes and mistakes later on.

CASE STUDY (8)

Veronica Irons, one of the partners at the John Street Health Centre, invited Cathy Colby, the new practice manager, to her home for a meal to talk over Cathy's unhappiness after only a few weeks in the practice. They discussed the practice, its values, its problems, and Cathy's role as Veronica saw it. Veronica suggested that Cathy had the same conversation with each of the partners, and she undertook to talk through with the others a proper induction programme for Cathy.

At the next partners' meeting, the partners agreed with Cathy that each partner should go over with her their area of responsibility. They suggested useful journals and books for Cathy to read, and arranged then and there to introduce her properly to the bank manager, the accountant, the FHSA general manager and the local pharmacists. She also had a list of contacts she needed to get to know – the Medical Audit Advisory Group (MAAG) chairman and administrator, as well as the local medical adviser, the administrator of the local RCGP faculty, the secretary of the local medical committee (LMC), the nurse managers, as well as the local pathology laboratory and X-ray services.

She applied to join the local branch of AHCPA and the practice agreed to pay her subscription and allow her time to attend local meetings and courses, including that organization's annual conference.

Cathy arranged to see all the staff at a meeting with Bill String, the senior partner, at which they explained the aims and tasks of Cathy's job and what the partners expected of her. She answered questions from the staff. Some of these surprised her, such as 'Will we have to clock in?', 'Will we have to wear uniforms?', 'Will any of us be made redundant?', 'What can you teach us about receptionist work when you have never done it?' and so on. It was clear that there had been a lot of misapprehension on all sides.

The meeting was difficult at times and Bill was astonished at the depth of feeling amongst staff because they had not been kept informed by the partners about what was going on. However Cathy now had some clues about where to get answers to questions, and what questions to ask. She felt that she could consult the partners without seeming to be a nuisance or a fool, and that the ice had been broken with the staff. She could set about getting to know them all individually. She felt much more able to attack the tasks facing her, and to help the others, both staff and partners, to do their part in the work of the practice.

Terms and conditions of employment

Although employers are not legally required to provide the written statement of terms and conditions of employment – commonly called the written contract – immediately the employee starts work (*see* Chapter 2), the induction process is helped by having on paper the details of employment and the rules and regulations relating to work at the practice. Explaining these in detail during the first few days may confuse the new employee; they are after all coping with a new environment and a new job. Within the first few weeks, however, the written statement should be discussed. This discussion should include the rules and regulations of the practice, such things as the standard of dress and personal use of the telephone, and – very importantly – the practice's disciplinary rules and procedures (*see* Chapter 7).

There may be some issues which need to be discussed within hours of the new person starting. For instance, even if the issue of patient confidentiality has been covered at the interview, it is important to repeat it and ensure that the employee is fully aware of the consequences of any breaches.

Health and safety

Ironically, health and safety training is much neglected in general practice and should be dealt with at the earliest stage. The implied terms of the contract of employment, which encompass health and safety, have been discussed in Chapter 2, and these implied terms come under civil law. However, employers have additional responsibilities under the Health and Safety at Work Act 1974, and subsequent regulations, and these duties come under criminal law.

Without going into great detail here, there are three areas all staff need to be aware of as soon as they join the practice:

- what to do in case of an accident – the procedure and the location of the accident book and first-aid box
- what to do in case of a fire

- the practice's Health and Safety Policy Statement, which is required by law. The local Environmental Department and the Health and Safety Executive (*see* Appendix C) will provide advice and guidance.

It is not sufficient merely to ask employees to read the policy and the relevant procedures. The employer is bound to ensure that the employee is aware of their own responsibilities. A short questionnaire after training is helpful to reinforce the position and check understanding. Figure 3.1 gives an example.

John Street Health Centre
Health and Safety Questionnaire

Now you have been trained, can you answer the following questions?

- Who is responsible for health and safety?
- What does the continuous sound of the fire alarm mean to you?
- In case of evacuation, where do you assemble?
- If you found something unsafe, what would you do?
- If you had any sort of accident, however small, what should you do?
- How should used needles be disposed of and what are the dangers?

Figure 3.1: Sample questionnaire to be completed after training

Employees should be asked to sign a form stating that they have received health and safety training in the required areas. This complies with the law and ensures that the employee is aware of the importance the practice places on health and safety.

The management style and structure

The management style of a practice will soon become apparent to all new staff (Prentice, 1990). This style can be characterized by answers that a practice would give to the following questions:

1 *Are mistakes tolerated and viewed as an opportunity to learn or*

are they viewed as personal failures and evidence of incompetence? This question is of particular importance to new staff. Any new job takes time to learn and mistakes are inevitable, and a feeling that reprimands will follow errors does more to undermine the confidence of a new employee than any other single factor.

2 *Is the practice characterized by consensus and co-operation, or by fear and divisiveness?* It is worthwhile explaining to new staff the role that staff play in the running of the practice. If decisions are discussed with staff and if they are regularly consulted, then it is important to say so. The willingness of the partners and practice manager to listen to suggestions from staff for improving the practice is vital and will encourage staff both to attend and participate in practice meetings. However, if the practice does not intend to take notice of staff suggestions in these circumstances, then it is better not to raise expectations falsely.

3 *Does everyone know the scope of their authority?* For instance, is it the receptionist or the practice manager who decides to add 'extras' onto the appointment list? If it is the receptionist, when will she be told that she can make such a decision?

4 *How is supervision exercised and what are the scope and main duties of the other practice team members?* Giving new staff copies of the up-to-date job descriptions of colleagues, including the practice manager's, may be important.

5 *Does the practice have a development plan and mission statement which can be used to explain to new staff the priorities and interests of the practice?*

6 *Does the practice undertake research activities, or are the partners involved in general practice education?*

7 *If the practice is involved in vocational training, what does being a training practice mean for the practice and the new employee?* It may be important to spend time outlining the process of general practice training to a newcomer.

8 *What is the role of the trainee in the practice and what role should the staff play in his or her training?*

9 *Who do the practice nurses report to and what is the relationship between the practice manager and the practice nurse?* The lack of induction training given to practice nurses is a current issue in general practice. The clinical induction training is often addressed but the non-clinical induction needs of new practice nurses is often ignored. General practice has a unique structure and practices differ from each other. Working in a hospital is very different from

working in a practice and new nurses, as much as any new member of staff, need to be inducted into the organization.

10 *Is the manager to whom the new recruit is accountable, accessible and available?* The new employee will, at this stage, not have had the time to establish new relationships within the practice and will indeed be alone. Ensuring that the person's manager or mentor is available will prevent the feeling that access to help is difficult and that requests for time are a constant imposition.

Internal promotions

Chapter 1 addressed the issue of introducing the internal candidate to their new promoted post. Obviously current staff who are promoted need a far shorter induction programme than staff who are new to the practice. However, all new jobs require some form of learning and any newly promoted internal candidate will be particularly keen to do well in the eyes of her colleagues.

Example 3.1

Elizabeth was promoted from being a full-time receptionist to being senior receptionist, supervising a well established team of three full-time and four part-time receptionists and a records clerk. She was young, enthusiastic and ambitious. She saw the possibility of a career in management, and the practice manager saw her as a possible successor. She was therefore very anxious to do well, and conscious of the expectations and pressures upon her.

Everyone was very aware of her lack of experience, and a number of the staff were surprisingly sensitive to the difficulties involved in a young, inexperienced member of staff supervising those older in years and experience with whom she had recently been on a par. One or two of the older staff were less sympathetic. The partners paid for her to go on an AMSPAR training course, and sent her to spend time with a senior receptionist at the neighbouring practice who was doing a similar job.

On her first full week in the job, under guidance from the practice manager, she saw each of the staff individually and

---

talked to them about their views on how the work was distributed and carried out, and what ideas they had for improving the processes. Without giving any promises she listened and took on board their ideas.

She took all their ideas and her own to the practice manager and between them they sorted out those that could work and those that would not. She then held a meeting with the receptionists and discussed the changes that could and should be made. That was the first of the regular weekly meetings they had at lunchtime over coffee and sandwiches. The staff liked her approach and consultative style, and the way she had taken their ideas and developed them. The partners and practice manager appreciated the way she had consulted up and down before making any changes. Above all she felt supported by the partners and practice manager, was clear about her role, felt trained and equipped, and saw some early successes to establish her in her new position.

Doing a completely new job is mentally exhausting and mistakes will be made, so a practice might consider allowing the new promotee to retain some tasks from their old job. A combination of the familiar, where the person can feel at ease and competent, with the new tasks and responsibilities can do much to maintain and increase their level of confidence.

Example 3.2

Leslie, the full-time accounts clerk at a practice, was promoted to be senior receptionist. She asked if she could keep the accounts work at which she was excellent, and the partners, who had no practice manager, reluctantly agreed. At first the receptionists still saw her as the accounts clerk because she was surrounded by figures on two afternoons a week. When she was not dealing with figures, however, they found that she was gradually gaining understanding of their jobs and had ideas for improving their ways of working.

The partners still saw her as the accounts clerk too, but also found that her competence in that role was not impaired by her new duties. They transferred the trust they had for her financial abilities to her supervisory ones. They found after

two months that she was a great success. Leslie herself felt
confident with the practice accounts and, because she
continued to have success in that area, the slowness of learning
the new job did not reduce her self-confidence. She found that
she had time to do both jobs as she only gradually took up the
senior receptionist role. After two or three months she felt
confident enough, and had sufficient new ideas she wanted to
try out in the reception area that she persuaded the partners
to employ a junior to train in accounts.

Good induction need not be costly, whereas ineffective induction can
prove expensive in the long term, and undermine all the efforts to
recruit the right person. It can provide a valuable baseline for and make
a major contribution to maintaining a motivated and well developed
workforce. The other factors involved in motivation and development
are explored in the next chapter.

4   How to Motivate and Develop Staff

HAVING appointed the perfect candidate, overcome the legal hurdles in agreeing a contract, and then appropriately inducted the person in their new post, the next management task is to ensure that the new appointee is properly motivated and so can develop within the job. The difference between successful and unsuccessful organizations can depend on, and largely rests with, the people who work in them. Highly motivated and committed staff can turn a complaint into a public relations exercise or a potential disaster into a solvable problem. They can also help positively to develop and improve the quality of the work of the organization. However, the reverse applies as well. Regardless of the location, quality of the premises or the sophistication of the administrative systems in place, a badly motivated workforce and incompetent management (the two are usually bedfellows) will ensure that the organization will fail to realize its potential.

Addressing the motivation of the practice team is consequently of fundamental importance to the management of a practice. Indeed it should be at the forefront of any decisions which impact on staff and the management style adopted by the leaders in the practice.

Box 4.1 summarizes the factors that help staff improve their performance and the performance of the practice.

Box 4.1: Motivating factors
- Recognition and praise, when deserved, from patients and colleagues.
- Consistency and fairness.
- Clarity of goals and the purpose of the job.
- Clarity of the expectations of performance.
- An atmosphere where flexibility and innovation is encouraged.
- Being consulted.
- Being part of a successful team.
- Knowing what constitutes success.
- Pressure, within reason.

- Variety of work.
- Challenging work.
- Working with people who are supportive.
- Having the authority and respect effectively to carry out the job.
- Learning new skills.
- Loyalty and support from staff.
- A sense of belonging.
- Encouragement.
- Achievements and efforts being valued and appreciated.

Recognition and praise

People need praise and recognition to motivate them – but such praise should only be given when deserved.

Example 4.1

A new practice manager was appointed who had limited experience in motivating staff. However, she was aware from her own experiences that staff were motivated when they receive praise for the work they do. During her first few weeks in the job, she ensured that the staff received such recognition regularly by way of phrases such as 'Well done, that's a really good job you have done' and 'I am impressed by the way you handled that awkward patient'. The staff were pleased that their new manager seemed to appreciate the work they did and they responded positively.

However, this management behaviour continued indiscriminately. Soon the practice manager noticed that the praise and compliments which previously were greeted with appreciation were being received with indifference. Indeed, when one receptionist administered first aid to a collapsed patient, the receptionist's response to the manager's 'Well done' was merely to say 'Look, you don't really mean it, so why say it?' and to walk away.

The manager in Example 4.1 failed to realize that compliments thrown around like confetti soon lose their value, and the respect of staff for the manager is damaged. People know when they have made a special effort, demonstrated a difficult skill, or have attained a high level of expertise, but compliments for normal everyday work soon lose their currency.

Recognizing exceptional work should be discussed so that the employee knows that their manager is fully aware of the effort or difficulties they faced in achieving success. It is a common mistake to confine recognition to a successful result; often exceptionally hard work or a lot of stress may lead only to failure. Confining recognition to successes will demotivate staff, as they will fail to see the purpose of extra effort if success is not guaranteed.

Challenging work

Giving demanding work and allowing staff to work under pressure can boost confidence. Keeping back all the challenging and responsible tasks (which are usually the most interesting ones) can also imply a lack of confidence and trust in employees.

Example 4.2

When a new practice manager was appointed she understood from the job description that she was expected to manage all the financial aspects of the practice, reporting as appropriate to the partners. However, it was clear very early on that not all the partners were happy with this in reality, and she found it difficult to obtain the basic data to make a start. One of the partners had always undertaken all the financial duties of the practice, and he revealed when challenged at a partnership meeting that he felt such a responsibility, which included PAYE calculations, could not be left to the practice manager. Indeed he felt that no member of staff should be privy to the partners' personal incomes. He was a perfectionist and believed no other person in the practice was able to achieve the standards of accuracy he reached. In any case, he enjoyed the work and did it in his own time!

The other partners were not prepared to support the practice manager and provoke a row within the partnership. The

---

practice manager therefore felt excluded, which damaged her motivation; she also continued to find it difficult to do her job without having access to the practice accounts.

Effective delegation is an art that can be learned, and some simple rules are set out in Box 4.2.

Box 4.2: Rules of delegation
- Never do work which others can do.
- Think carefully about why you are delegating.
- Set out the process of control and review.
- Delegate the whole job.
- Delegate adequate resources.
- Ensure complete understanding.
- Criticize only in private.
- Ask others what you can delegate to them.
- Retain responsibility for the results.
- Use delegation to criticize your own performance.

Source: RCGP (1986)

First of all it is vital to be sure why a task or responsibility is being delegated at all, and what that delegation is meant to achieve, so that the staff can understand the purpose too. Secondly there must be the appropriate resources available (*see* Box 4.3).

Box 4.3: Resources that may be necessary
- Time.
- Equipment.
- Space.
- Access to information and guidance.
- Training.

This preparatory work needs to be followed up with clear communication and consultation (*see* Box 4.4). This is a crucial phase. Delegation goes wrong most often because communication has not been clear.

Box 4.4: The components of communication
- Explaining why you are delegating the task.
- Explaining why you selected the person.
- Clarifying what you expect and what criteria will be used to assess the success of the results.
- Stating whether or not there is a time limit for completion.

Frequently what managers say may be misunderstood, so it is vital to look at the clarity of instructions. A delegator needs to be satisfied that he or she has the listener's attention and that instructions are explained clearly. Then the frequency with which instructions are misunderstood or misinterpreted can be used as a good indication of staff morale (Stewart, 1979).

The task or responsibility must be delegated to the most appropriate person, with the relationship between competence and confidence being taken into account. The most confident staff may not necessarily be the most competent and vice versa. It is easy to delegate work to the most willing volunteer and to ignore the most reluctant (Turner, 1992).

It is important to seek out alternative views on how the job could be done and, where possible, to allow the delegatee to plan and implement the work. It is also worth agreeing what sort of supervision is needed and wanted, and the way the work will be reviewed. People appreciate being given the responsibility for a job, but this is undermined if managers 'hover around' or retain part of the task unnecessarily.

If work is delegated unskilfully, staff tend to view it (often quite justifiably) as 'dumping'. The impression is that managers are giving them tasks which they themselves do not want to spend time on, rather than demonstrating trust and confidence in their employees or giving them the opportunity to develop.

If the delegation has been carried out skilfully, and it still goes wrong, then the delegator has to accept that they selected the wrong person to do the task. This admission needs to be made diplomatically to the employee concerned, and it is important to allow the person to save face and to maintain a sense of self-esteem. A discussion of this needs to be conducted in private. Merely announcing the decision to reclaim the task, particularly if this is done in front of other staff, is poor management and a sure way not only of demotivating the person concerned but also of generating an unwillingness in all staff to volunteer or accept new work.

Example 4.3

A partner asked the practice manager to set up a practice library as they were aiming to become a training practice in the near future. She was pleased to do so, and set about researching the subject, talking to colleagues in other practices and getting reading lists from the RCGP and the local postgraduate institute library. She made a budget and put a paper together for the next practice meeting.

At that meeting, when they reached that item, the partner who had delegated the task to her announced that he had sent a list of required books to the local medical bookshop, had arranged for the practice to receive certain additional journals, and had arranged for the librarian at the local large group practice to come and tell the partners how to set up the new library, and how much it would cost. He completely ignored the fact that he had asked the manager to do any work, and she felt undermined and deflated. All her enthusiasm for the library project disappeared.

Often the development potential of giving challenging work to staff is not fully exploited. The work may be completed but nothing happens as a result. For the practice to gain fully, and to foster staff motivation, the third stage of delegation – that of monitoring the results – needs to be implemented. This serves to create an environment where people feel able to learn from their experiences.

Example 4.4

A receptionist was asked to develop a new repeat-prescribing system that would take full account of the practice's prescribing policies and use the full potential of the computer software available. After three weeks' hard work and thought, she produced a simple but effective system which was implemented forthwith.

After two months the practice manager had an interview with the receptionist and discussed with her whether the results of

---

the new system were what the practice expected, in what ways it was even more effective than expected, and in what ways it failed to meet expectations. They discussed the ways in which it might be further improved and then discussed what the receptionist had learned from doing the task and achieving the results.

The receptionist was so encouraged by the interest that her system had generated that she suggested she spent more time and energy looking at the way the appointment system itself worked and what opportunities there were to computerize that.

Any venture which involves understanding people and trusting them involves risk. However, by not taking the risk of delegating, managers may unwittingly take the bigger risk of wasting resources and even, ultimately, losing the staff they should be developing and retaining (Melton and Long, 1990).

CASE STUDY (9)

Cathy Colby, the new practice manager at the John Street Health Centre, raised the whole question of staff development with the partners at a formal weekly meeting soon after she arrived at the practice. She used an example from a week or two earlier which showed how poor delegation and misuse of staff had prevented staff development. At that time Cathy herself was still feeling insecure and not sure of the practice's protocols.

The incident had occurred over an urgent need to take on temporary staff to assist in the inputting of data into the computer. Betty Waters (the senior receptionist) and Cathy had convinced Tom Cutter (the partner responsible) of the importance of recruiting temporary help, and they agreed that Tom and Cathy would put the case to the next partners' meeting. It was urgent because the staff were becoming discouraged that it took so long to input data into the computer.

Unfortunately the partners decided at the last minute to bring the meeting forward to a day which clashed with a long-awaited hospital appointment Cathy had arranged to deal with a minor but persistent ear problem. She could not alter the appointment at such short notice, and the only item of major concern on the agenda was the creation of a temporary clerk post. She hoped that Tom could handle it well enough on his own. On the morning of the meeting Tom suggested that he would be happier if he had Betty at the meeting, to help put the case in Cathy's absence. He told Cathy that Betty was quite used to speaking at the partners' meetings and would have no worries about it.

Cathy felt that Betty was rather nervous of the doctors, but that this might be an opportunity to increase her confidence. Betty reluctantly agreed to attend the meeting and was reassured by Cathy's assertion that Tom would be handling the item and that she would be taking a back seat. Cathy finally added that Betty might be needed to back up Tom, and said: 'It is important to get across to the partners the seriousness of the situation and convince them of the need for more investment in this area. You might find it helpful to write down all the reasons why we need extra help, if only temporarily. Here are the financial implications so far as I can work them out at the moment, though of course I've not had a chance yet to look into the whole of the resource needs of the practice. I've calculated the costs both with reimbursement and without. Is that all clear? Just do your best.'

Betty nodded in unhappy agreement, and as she went out Cathy added 'We are all relying on you, Betty.' After the meeting and when Cathy got back from her hospital appointment, she called Betty in and asked how it went. 'Well, the best I could get was overtime for existing staff up to 19 hours a week for four weeks.' Cathy replied, 'Well, that is disappointing. Clearly the partners did not understand the situation. Didn't Tom make the case?' 'No,' said Betty. 'When the item came, he said that as you couldn't be there I was going to put the case on your behalf.' 'It was not my case,' expostulated Cathy. 'He's the one who wants the data on more quickly.' 'What exactly did you say?' 'Well, I gave them the costings you had prepared and said we were overworked and that I was worried that all our items of service are not being properly claimed. But I couldn't say by how much because I hadn't thought of that in time. Dr String told me off for being negative, and said that my job was to lead the receptionist team in as positive and upbeat a way as possible. I felt so awful I shut up then.'

'So you see,' Cathy said to the partners when she had finished the story, 'between us we managed to ruin a senior member of staff's confidence in herself, her manager, and the partners, as well as making her feel she was incompetent, negative and a fool, and letting down everyone including the staff.' All the partners nodded thoughtfully.

Consistency and fairness

Consistency and fairness are fundamental to motivating staff. Allocating work, operating the salary structure, applying terms and conditions of employment, handling disciplinary issues and promoting staff are some of the issues which can test a manager's consistency of approach.

Staff do not expect to be treated equally in all aspects of work – for instance, receptionists do not expect to earn the same as practice managers and, equally, less experienced staff do not expect to have the same level of work delegated to them as to the more experienced. Differentiation between employees is not only inevitable but necessary for the effective management of the practice. However it is important to be sure that *all* concerned (not just the recipient) are aware of the reasons behind such differentials.

Many practices make the mistake of assuming that staff will keep their salaries confidential. This is rarely true. Therefore if there are anomalies and inconsistences in staff pay, the practice should address this as a matter of priority. Staff may tolerate a member of staff earning more than others, if such a person is more experienced and skilled. Staff, quite rightly, have difficulty in accepting anomalies where the most competent, willing and skilled personnel earn lower salaries than less able employees.

Linking pay to performance is covered in more detail in Chapter 6 but it is worth underlining here that if staff are paid on a higher grade to others, then it is important that they are actually and demonstrably undertaking responsibilities of a higher level. This can do much to prevent resentment.

Clarity of purpose and expectations of performance

A well managed practice is a practice where people are not only aware of the overall purpose of their individual jobs but also how their jobs fit into the overall purpose of the practice. In other words, people need to feel that their jobs are meaningful. People can only work as a team, as opposed to merely a collection of individuals, if they feel that their jobs are important to the very essence of the organization. If a practice's overall purpose is continually to improve the quality of care patients receive, everyone in the practice needs to know this and to be aware of how their individual jobs play a real part in achieving that purpose (Turrill, 1986; Handy, 1987).

Receptionists need to know that the quality of patient care is very much dependent on the work of the receptionist, from dealing with the initial enquiry, welcoming the patient, arranging an appointment, to the efficiency with which all the other administrative tasks of their jobs are undertaken. Misfiled medical records, or an unhelpful attitude towards patients, affect the quality of care patients receive. Doctors can be very guilty of assuming that the time spent in the consulting room is the only criterion by which the practice is judged. This assumption can undermine staff and prevents employees from operating as a team (Drury, 1990).

CASE STUDY (10)

After a month in post as the new practice manager at the John Street Health Centre, Cathy Colby felt the need to be more specific about what she wanted to do and how she wanted to be judged. She was still unclear about what the partnership expected of her and the staff (beyond day-to-day protocols about interrupting surgeries for telephone calls), and what she understood of the practice's stated aims.

The partners were very pleased with the way Cathy was doing, but were still surprised at the amount of time they were still spending on what they felt were non-clinical issues. They all felt that the general level of management in the practice had been raised by Cathy's excellent financial and personnel expertise. Clearly therefore there was still more to do in communicating and motivating.

Cathy was not aware of the partners' confidence in her, because day-to-day matters still went wrong and she spent a great deal of time sorting them out. She felt that the doctors were still not sure whether they wanted a robotic administrator, or someone to help in strategic management.

She asked for a review meeting, which she arranged with some difficulty and to which in the event only two partners, Veronica Irons and Stephen Wood, came. Cathy had set down in draft short-, medium- and long-term targets. In the short term she aimed to improve the practice as an employer by instituting proper contracts of employment for all staff, setting up and publishing disciplinary and grievance procedures, revising all the terms and conditions of service such as sick and maternity leave to conform to modern employer practice, monitoring recruitment procedures (particularly to ensure that no discrimination was creeping in), and looking at ways of improving the remuneration package and motivators.

All this, she explained, was a background to looking at ways of improving productivity by improving the motivation of the staff. She now knew the reasons each member of the team went to work and why each of them did their particular job. All their reasons were different and so different motivators were needed.

She also wanted to change her office to a more private room away from the hurly burly of the reception to underline that she was not dealing with the day-to-day matters; the senior receptionist did that. It would also give her the peace and quiet she needed both to speak to people and to draw up the systems and papers needed to get these plans off the ground.

She offered these short-term targets as her initial assessment of what was needed to motivate both her and the team. Next she needed clear aims and objectives from the partnership to assess her longer-term targets. What was the timetable for decisions on fundholding, for instance, and did they want her to take over lead responsibility for investigating it and bringing the systems and data up to date? What were the current targets for moving to new premises? There was a site available but they had not discussed it fully. She felt they would lose the opportunity soon. Did they want to move to new premises before fundholding or after? Did they want to expand the partnership or stay the same size? Did they want to build a surgery large enough to house other services such as counselling and physiotherapy? Did the FHSA want to use new premises – was there any negotiation there for the renting of a part of new premises? Did they want to take on minor surgery? What was their aim in relation to being a training practice again?

Decisions on all these areas were needed to provide clear objectives to all the staff and help everyone decide on their priorities. Veronica and Stephen talked all these issues through with Cathy, but when they spoke to Bill String, the senior partner, he was horrified at the idea of introducing written terms and conditions of service for staff, particularly grievance procedures which he thought would provoke a rash of complaints about individual partners.

Cathy assured the partners that she would bring papers on these issues to partnership meetings as she prepared them. However, she made it clear that the wider issues of the practice's overall direction and policy could not be subsumed within narrower issues of discipline, if the motivation and development of the team was to be sustained.

Learning new skills

Learning new skills, whether within the practice or on external courses, is fundamental to any organization which employs new staff and which is undergoing change. General practice is no stranger to change, and the training needs of managers and staff have grown in the last few years. The days of 'sitting by Nellie' and viewing the management of the practice on a 'buggins turn' basis are gone. The training needs of staff are addressed in more detail in Chapter 7.

Financial incentives

What is most interesting about any list of motivators is the absence of money. It does play a part in motivation in that it can act as a demotivator if recipients feel financially undervalued or if they perceive anomalies in the pay structure disadvantageous to themselves. However, the relationship between money and motivation has to be seen in its proper context, and the demands of management now require a more sophisticated approach to motivating staff.

Role models

Role modelling is an important aspect of the manager's work. If a doctor fails to say 'good morning' and does not treat staff with respect, then he or she cannot expect the staff to be ambassadors for the practice. The standards expected of staff in the performance of their duties and their relations with others are led and reinforced by the behaviour of the managers, both clinical and non-clinical, in the practice. Expecting staff to follow the decisions made at partners' meetings is unrealistic if the partners themselves do not adhere to such decisions.

A person's immediate manager is the biggest single influence on his or her effectiveness, happiness at work, morale and personal growth. Everyone with managerial responsibilities therefore must undertake an active role in developing their staff and be aware of the role-model function they play in their relationships with their employees.

Recognizing and addressing the fact that peoples' knowledge, skills, capabilities, motivation and value do not develop automatically is a crucial management skill. People need to be cultivated, nurtured and cared for in a planned and considered fashion. They need to be empowered to achieve their potential in their jobs as well as possible through recognizing and fulfilling their training and developmental needs. The next chapter addresses how to manage that process.

5 How to Train Staff

This chapter addresses the management activities and skills necessary to meet the training needs of all those working in the practice. Timely and appropriate training is often the key to the process of organizational growth and development. It is so important that practices may need to create a partnership mechanism to ensure that training has the appropriate priority and focus throughout the practice, for doctors, nurses, and administrative, clerical and receptionist staff. This mechanism might for instance be the designation of a partner to be responsible for education and training. Indeed the new Trade Union Reform and Employment Rights Bill 1993 entitles all employees who work for an organization employing 20 or more staff the right to receive a statement as to how the organization's training affects them.

The purpose of training

Managers have a primary task, which pervades all management activity, and that is to use human resources effectively. Research has shown that most people operate on 40% of their potential (Harvey-Jones, 1988). People who work at 60% of their potential are doing very well. Getting from 40% to 60% is not easy but whatever methods are used to motivate and stimulate staff, nothing will work unless employees have the knowledge and skills to do their jobs effectively. Managers, be they clinical or lay, need to ensure that all members of the practice team are equipped with that necessary knowledge, understanding and skills to undertake their part in the practice's work in a manner and to a standard that delivers the quality and quantity of care defined by the practice's aims.

No organization can honestly say that there is no room for training. Well trained staff are cost-effective, and training needs met within the practice are usually cheaper than when they are met through attending outside courses. However, not all the practice's training needs will be able to be met within the practice.

There is another, more mundane, reason for addressing training, which is of course linked to the above, and that is that FHSAs and Health Boards in Scotland are now taking a far greater interest in practice staff training and training qualifications. This interest, particularly if there are financial implications, should not be confined to attendance at courses but will also embrace the training being done within the practice.

The main purposes of training are summarized in Box 5.1.

Box 5.1: The purposes of training
- To improve the effectiveness of individuals in their current jobs and thereby enhancing their motivation.
- To facilitate change.
- To promote high standards and good practice.

The elements of training

The principal tasks of any manager's training role are:

- to identify accurately the training needs of the practice
- to select the most appropriate method of meeting these needs
- to select the most cost-effective method
- to prioritize training needs
- to provide in-house training
- to evaluate training.

Identifying training needs

To identify training needs effectively, a manager must have a clear perception of the practice's aims and future plans as well as detailed knowledge of the gaps between current and desired performance. Certain questions need to be asked in order to identify the gap between what is current and what is desired performance. Here are three examples.

1 A person may be performing well now but what will their training needs be in six months' time?

2 Is the practice introducing or updating a computer system? Is the practice going to apply for fundholding?

3 Does the practice intend to become a training practice?

Identifying training needs in advance of change is an important factor in managing change successfully.

In addition, a need to look at training can be provoked by specific events such as the induction of new staff (*see* Chapter 3), or where changes in the practice may require practice staff to assume new tasks and roles, or require them to adopt different attitudes. The skills and knowledge requirements of any such proposed changes are easier to identify than the attitudinal changes that may be needed, but they must also be addressed and are discussed later in this chapter.

Example 5.1

When the partners of a practice first introduced computers they identified the training needs of the staff only in terms of operating the computer. They did not address the anxieties some of the staff had about new technology generally.

A training programme was arranged and the computer supplier duly arrived to instruct the staff in the computer's operation. This training was clear and professionally delivered.

For three of the members of staff though this training was a waste of time. Their anxieties were such that much of the instruction was not heeded – their minds were focused on their fears about making fools of themselves in front of the other staff, wiping out the data, and their belief that the whole area of new technology was too complicated for them.

Consequently, some of their fears were realized. Their inattention during the training session meant that they were the least competent computer users and one of them did indeed manage to lose a large quantity of data. Further training was clearly needed to deal with lost confidence and resistance to change.

This example demonstrates how a practice set out a training programme for staff to adapt to a new skill, but failed to address the attitudes held by staff to learning the new skill. Identifying the training needs dictated by change is often easier than identifying the training needs required when there is not an obvious change. This is because new events will require new, rather than improved, skills. The example above demonstrates that even something as straightforward as the introduction of a new computer needs careful thought to match the training to skills, knowledge and attitude.

It does not however anticipate and therefore manage the attitudinal changes needed. This can be more pointedly demonstrated over the issue of internal promotion (*see* Chapters 1 and 3). For instance, there has often been a lack of appreciation of the training needs of a new practice manager, who has been promoted from within. Being responsible for the work of others requires different skills to being merely responsible for one's own work. In addition, the training needs of practice staff to accept and support the new manager have often been ignored.

The job description

Identifying training needs cannot be carried out in isolation. The starting point is the job description. Unless a job has been described and defined, identifying the training needs of the job holder would be like writing a shopping list without knowing what is in the pantry! Job descriptions are a fundamental tool of management and play a role in recruitment and selection (*see* Chapter 1), the motivation of staff (*see* Chapter 4) and performance appraisal (*see* Chapter 6) as well as training.

The job description should preferably include the knowledge and skills demanded of each task, as analysing these requirements of the post is essential in identifying training needs. Chapter 1 describes how this process is completed.

The training interview

Once the job description has been designed, the job holder needs to be interviewed. This part of the process is crucial as presenting the employee with a *fait accompli* of their training needs will do little to maintain confidence in the practice's training scheme or its management. Also people often feel threatened by training and may perceive a discussion of needs as an admission of weakness. Explaining what is being done and its underlying purpose will do much to allay anxieties.

Generally employees themselves can offer valuable contributions and observations.

The job holder will have to make a very real contribution to assessing their own needs if they are to feel committed to undertaking any training. However, when a training exercise is introduced, more ambitious staff may see it as a green light to undertake expensive and not necessarily relevant training. Therefore expectations must be realistic and even where genuine training needs have been identified it is important that the employee is aware that not all such needs can be met. After all, the resources of the practice will be a major factor in determining training priorities.

It is useful to give each employee a series of questions to consider before the interview. These are set out in Box 5.2.

Box 5.2: Questions for a training interview
- What do I need to know in order to do my job?
- What do I need to know to do my job in the future, as it progresses? (This question may not be applicable to all staff.)
- What do I need to know for my own satisfaction?
- Which parts of my job take up the most time?
- Which parts of my job do I find the most worrying or difficult?
- What in my job would I like to do better?
- Are there any factors which hinder me in carrying out my job?
- Do I have skills which I could impart to other members of staff which would help them in their jobs?

The training interview is similar to the recruitment interview (*see* Chapter 1). All interviews are controlled conversations with a purpose, but the training interview can assume a less formal atmosphere than most other work-related interviews. Nevertheless, anxieties will be experienced by some staff so it is important to follow the rules of interviewing to establish rapport and explain the purpose of the meeting.

One of the aims of the training interview is to help the interviewee identify their own training needs. In any exercise involved in gleaning information skilful questioning and listening techniques are vital. The two are interrelated and are discussed in detail in Chapters 1 and 6.

A training interview can fail if:

- the purpose of the interview is not explained
- too many closed, leading or multiple types of questions are asked
- the interviewer does not listen and talks too much
- the interviewee is ridiculed
- training is wrongly identified as a remedy for problems which actually require different solutions
- the interview is allowed to drift into a grievance or disciplinary interview (*see* Chapter 5)
- expectations are raised which cannot be fulfilled.

The interview should end with a summary of the agreed training needs and an indication of which of those needs can be met, how they will be met, and the timing.

Once the interviews have been completed, the information gained must be collated, analysed, prioritized and used to form the practice's training programme. The programme need not be elaborate, but should form a summary of the practice's training needs, as set out in Box 5.3.

Box 5.3: Practice training programme
Who needs to be trained.
What they need to be trained in or for (ie the training subject).
How they will be trained (ie the training method).
When they will be trained.

Meeting the training needs

The skill of matching needs to the most appropriate training method involves knowledge of the resources available inside and outside the practice. There are a number of suitable learning methods.

Methods of learning

'Sitting by Nellie'

This method is generally used for induction and involves little extra effort (*see* Chapter 3). However it has a number of drawbacks; Nellie may be a poor role model and bad habits are learnt as well as good. Just listening for several days or hours and then suddenly having to do the full job, before all the questions have been answered or all the tasks covered, may make the learner feel very exposed.

Small-group learning

In small-group learning, each member can contribute as well as listen and can thereby acquire knowledge, interpersonal skills and new attitudes. The group must be led, but unobtrusively. Box 5.4 sets out the main benefits of small-group learning.

Box 5.4: Advantages of small-group learning
- solving problems (eg how can we reduce the waiting times for appointments?)
- changing attitudes (eg how can we get the senior staff to recognize their responsibilities for training staff?)
- obtaining commitment (eg how can we ensure that the staff accept the new working arrangements?)
- developing ideas (eg how can we use the principles of audit in the practice?)

Didactic teaching

Normally this takes the form of lectures but it can be used informally to impart knowledge on a one-to-one basis, usually in induction training, eg explaining the main terms and conditions of employment and the 'house' rules of the practice to a new employee.

Experiential learning

'Learning by doing' can be done on the job under supervision, by role play and video sessions. It is suitable for learning problem-solving skills.

Distance learning

Pioneer work has been done through the Open University (OU) and the RCGP (RCGP, 1985, 1986, 1987, 1989, 1990, 1992). Exercises and projects are given to students with the knowledge and information needed to undertake the tasks. This input is given in various ways – written, aurally (tape or radio), or visually (TV, videos). Students submit their work to tutors who mark, assess and return it. The OU offers the opportunity to meet tutors and to attend summer schools.

Audio-visual aids

These are programmes which consist of a video filmed in modular form accompanied by a booklet which contains reading material and exercises related to the modules in the film. Learning with these can be done in groups or individually.

Courses

Staff are trained away from the practice usually by a trainer from outside the practice. Courses can last from half a day to five days. There are also vocational courses where the trainee attends a local college on a regular basis – usually once a week in term time. Many courses offer recognized qualifications.

Given the size and resources of most practices not all of these methods may be suitable for practice staff. However some lend themselves very well to in-house training. All methods involve the general principles of learning set out in Box 5.5 and each method involves one, or more often more than one, training technique which are described in detail in Appendix E.

Box 5.5: Some general principles of learning
- Self-research aids learning.
- If specific learning goals are set, learning is more likely to occur.
- Where the relevance of the material to be learned is made clear, more learning is likely.
- Awareness by the teacher and the learner of the obstacles to the learner's ability to learn will help the learner to succeed.

- Learning is more likely where expectations of success are high than when they are low.
- Learning is aided by an environment in which one feels 'safe' to make mistakes.
- Regular feedback and checking during the learning process increase the amount of learning.
- Learning is more likely to occur if the material presented builds on the learner's current knowledge and skills.
- Where the learner is actively involved, more learning is likely to occur.

In addition, all training methods (except lectures) require interaction between the trainer and the learner. Identifying any barriers to learning, assessing previous knowledge and skills, checking on understanding, reflective questions and stimulating ideas all require sophisticated questioning techniques. The importance of these techniques applies in all interviewing and Appendix H gives further structured examples of questioning techniques.

Evaluating training

If training is to be worthwhile in terms of contributing to the overall purpose of the practice, then its value needs to be determined in the same way as any other function. The value needs to be expressed in terms of the benefit not only to the learner but also to the practice itself. Too often, feedback consists of a casual remark – 'it was a good course' or 'I learned a lot.' These and the many other variations have no real meaning as they are not related to any defined and understood standard.

Training, whether inside the practice or outside, costs money, time and effort on the part of many people; it should have an objective and be geared to the needs of the practice.

There are three ways of determining the value of training, and they are closely linked.

- Assessing. The learner assesses the value to them personally
- Costing. The actual financial costs are determined
- Evaluating. Does the training achieve its aims?

Assessing

Assessing the value of training is done either individually or in groups at the end of the session or course, and may include practical as well as intellectual aspects. It is standard practice to use an assessment form at the end of formal training sessions and courses and for very good reasons. Although such an assessment is immediate and does not allow time for reflection, it can provide valuable information in the following areas.

- Did the course/session meet the aims of the training?
- Was the level of subject treatment too advanced, satisfactory or too elementary?
- Was the course paced too slow, too fast or just right?
- Was the course too long, satisfactory or too short?
- What was the learning value of the course? Although it is not possible to assess this at an early stage the trainees' perceptions of the learning value of the course is valuable.
- Which training techniques are most effective? The techniques will encompass some or all of the following depending on the course subject:
  − talks
  − group discussions
  − exercises
  − role plays
  − case studies
  − training films.
- What is the overall impression of the method of presentation?
- Are there any topics that should have been included in or removed from the course?

In addition to providing valuable information to the practice this feedback highlights whether or not the trainees' own expectations of the course were met.

When analysing the assessment of learning activities there are a number of factors to be considered. Some people naturally mark generously while some are grudging in their assessments. If the trainer is the trainee's boss, fear of repercussions may inhibit the assessment. Similarly, if the trainer is known personally to the trainee, fear of offending may inhibit the assessment. As a result often the personality of the trainer is assessed rather than the learning value of the training.

Costing

Training can be a costly business and it is advisable to set an annual budget for training. This cannot be done unless the practice has some idea of the costs involved.

Outside courses

In addition to the course fee there is also the expense of materials, transport and accommodation. If staff have to cover for the absent employee and overtime is required then this too should be calculated, including costs for time off in lieu. Hiring temporary staff to cover the absence is an obvious expense.

Although it cannot be quantified, it is a good idea to offset some of the costs by asking the person being trained to report back to the practice on completion of the course. This can take the form of a short report or talk. This gives the message to the trainee that the practice views training seriously, it reinforces the training and, depending on the subject, can provide valuable knowledge to the practice.

In-house training

Calculating the costs of in-house training can be more difficult and often needs to be so detailed that it can become a cost in itself! One-off job instruction sessions and the occasional talk need only a cursory assessment. Major practice endeavours though, such as introducing an appraisal scheme (see Chapter 6), do need more detailed costings.

Obvious expenses would be the fees of outside speakers/trainers/consultants, but not so obvious would be the hourly rates of pay of those staff receiving the training, administrative and clerical costs.

It is important to cost training in order to work out its value for money. Moreover letting staff know the cost of training reinforces the investment the practice is making in the trainee.

Evaluating

Measuring the effectiveness of the training will provide information which will help to select future courses, increase the effectiveness of later or even current training, and provide proof of the training function's contribution to the practice which can be used to increase its influence. Evaluating training involves the setting of objectives which tie into the training aim. It will measure the extent of the learner's new knowledge and skills and how far the learner is putting it into practice.

Evaluating learning and performance during in-house training can take place at stages during the training or left until after the training has been completed. Job instruction would involve asking the trainee to demonstrate the new skill as each state of learning is completed.

Other methods of evaluating learning (by tests, quizzes, questionnaires etc) should be used with care. They can cause great anxiety to trainees and can actually inhibit learning.

Evaluating performance is usually more straightforward than evaluating learning. Performance traits which can be quantified, eg keyboard skills, are less common in general practice than those which can only be evaluated through observation and appraisal – eg management skills and the ability to deal with awkward patients.

However 'intangible' the skills that a person has been trained in, it is important to ensure that an objective has been set for the training (and this includes outside courses), that the trainee is aware of the objective, that some form of evaluation takes place and that the evaluation is discussed with the learner.

Conclusion

Identifying training needs and meeting them, as well as evaluating the effectiveness of the training delivered, are skills which are essential for any manager who is responsible for staff. No organization can survive without people who are confident and competent in the tasks they undertake. Well thought-out and professionally delivered training develops and motivates staff. It can help the practice retain good employees and improve those whose performance does not reach the desired standards. It demonstrates the practice's commitment to quality performance.

How to Appraise Staff

For employees to develop, it is crucial that they know how their performance is being assessed and what constitutes satisfactory performance. An effective appraisal system forms a central plank of any practice's quality control policy.

Why appraise?

The principal purpose of any formal system of appraisal is to aid the overall task of managing an organization, such as general practice, by helping staff to develop and perform to their full potential (Wilson and Cole, 1990). It is there to assist in the key areas of a manager's general responsibilities – planning, co-ordinating and monitoring of work within the practice (*see* Figure 6.1).

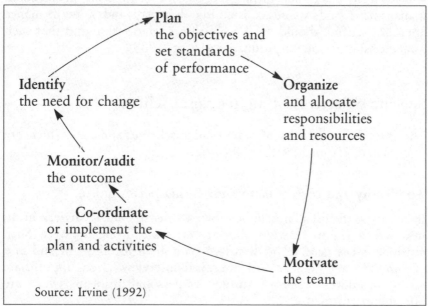

Source: Irvine (1992)

Figure 6.1: The management cycle

It offers the managers of a practice a formal and objective opportunity to assess how individual members of staff can best contribute to achieving the objectives of the practice; to identify areas where there is a duplication of effort; to pinpoint time spent on tasks which have now become obsolete; to identify and avoid any gaps in the work of the practice; and to create challenges for those individuals who are capable or have the potential to undertake new work.

Moreover it allows managers to check the accuracy of their perceptions of how well staff are performing and to ensure that these perceptions are shared with the individuals concerned. It is more comprehensive than the regular and invaluable but less structured daily assessments that managers undertake informally.

As in any management process, the purpose of an appraisal scheme must be well thought-out, clear, and properly communicated to all involved. If schemes attempt to fulfil different and/or conflicting requirements, then they can fail or cause dissatisfaction. For instance the most obvious areas for conflict can be found in schemes which are used to operate a salary review as well as to improve current performance – commonly known as performance related pay. People are unlikely to be honest if the recognition or revelation of a weakness will adversely affect their earnings. It is now recognized by professional management bodies and consultants that pay and a performance appraisal scheme should not have a direct relationship and that such a relationship is counterproductive (Hogg, 1988).

Specific objectives of an appraisal scheme

The intended objectives of a particular scheme, some of which are interrelated, can include the following.

To identify and correct factors impairing performance

It is very difficult, if not impossible, to discuss such barriers in an informal way, particularly if they are the fault of the employee. Such sensitive issues need to be discussed with great forethought and in a non-threatening manner. An appraisal interview is an appropriate setting to address issues of attitude or personal problems which are affecting performance.

Example 6.1
A receptionist was excellent at handling patients and was
extremely efficient at answering the telephone and making
appointments. However, she had an unfortunate habit of
shrugging her shoulders and treating the doctors with what
they saw as contempt. The partners were always complaining
about this to the practice manager who was nonplussed by the
problem. The setting up of an appraisal system enabled the
manager to have a formal structured meeting, with a formal
preliminary assessment of strengths and weaknesses set out
beforehand.

As a result the receptionist revealed that she was nervous of
doctors. As a small child she had had a very bad experience
leading her to relate doctors to pain and suffering. Her apparent
indifference bordering on offensiveness was in fact due to fear
and awe. The practice manager encouraged her to talk about it
and in turn made it explicit to the receptionist how her
apparent attitude affected others. They decided together on
some strategies for overcoming the attitudinal impact, and the
receptionist agreed at least to let the doctors know what was
behind her behaviour. As a result the doctors were able in turn
to modify their approach to her.

To develop a more collaborative style of management

Many of those practices which have successfully introduced an
appraisal scheme have identified improvement in communications and
relationship between the appraiser and appraisee as one of the major
benefits of the scheme.

Communication in organizations tends to follow the laws of gravity
– always going to the bottom! It is most useful to set up processes
which counteract this tendency and ensure, at the very least, a minimum level of communication both upwards and downwards in the
practice. An appraisal scheme can provide such a vehicle (Haman and
Williams, 1992).

To identify training and personal developmental needs

Training and developmental needs should ideally be identified from an overview of past performance and the planned future developments of the practice which will impact on the appraisee. Again an appraisal interview is the most suitable setting for such an exercise, as it can foster enthusiasm and commitment from the appraisee. Chapter 5 deals with training in more detail.

To reinforce present behaviour

As shown in Chapter 3, one motivator common to most people in work is the need for recognition. When this is given in a considered and sincere way, based on the evidence of a person's past performance and not merely on a general feeling that the person is operating effectively, the motivating potential of the recognition is greatly enhanced. An appraisal interview can alert managers to the need to recognize effort and success, and provide an opportunity to do without the complications of salary issues.

Benefits of an appraisal scheme

Benefits of appraisal may differ for the appraiser and the appraisee. For the practice, the areas that are likely to be improved by it are listed briefly in Box 6.1.

Box 6.1: Benefits of an appraisal scheme to the practice
- Effectiveness and efficiency.
- Corporate image.
- Team work.
- Evaluation of performance.
- Generation of new ideas.
- 'People' management skill.

Some of the benefits for the individual are set out in Box 6.2.

Box 6.2: Some benefits to the individual of an appraisal scheme
- Providing insight into personal motivation.
- Clarifying expectations.
- Improving effectiveness.
- Clarifying roles and boundaries between individual responsibilities.
- Reinforcing views of employing organization's fairness and consistency.
- Presenting opportunities to consider and formulate developmental plans.
- Allowing self-appraisal.
- Producing action plans.
- Helping to manage stress.

Example 6.2

A senior receptionist was very insecure in her own role. She tended therefore to be anxious about the way her receptionist colleagues carried out the tasks she delegated to them. In turn this raised their anxiety levels and tended to increase their mistakes.

At the appraisal interview she had with one receptionist, she brought up the level of mistakes as an issue of the receptionist's performance. The appraisee described how the senior receptionist had so harassed her when she had been trying to deal with a difficult phone call that she had made a mess of it. The patient on the other end had been upset, the relevant doctor had been angry, and the receptionist had been demoralized. The senior receptionist's anxious behaviour had created a drama out of a crisis because she had made her receptionist colleague perform below par.

The senior receptionist in turn felt able to reveal her anxiety levels and her reasons for putting pressure on others. Greater understanding was reached on both sides, which in due course led to changes of behaviour in everyone.

Example 6.2 shows how there are mutual benefits as well. Feedback is essential to the effective performance of any individual or any organization. The performance appraisal process helps objectivity in this evaluation process. It helps managers to judge and be seen to be judging fairly. The appraisal system can help affirm to the employee that their performance is effective and valued, as well as identifying areas which require improvement.

Example 6.3

A partner with responsibility for staff held an appraisal interview with the practice manager. They had had several informal exchanges in the corridor about the way she was developing the appointments system, but the practice manager had been a little anxious about the partners' views on the system. The appraisal interview was an opportunity in a detached and objective way to go through the detail of her feeling about the present system's strengths and weaknesses, to assess it and the way she had introduced it.

As a result she altered several elements and felt sufficiently encouraged to propose more variations, including some that affected the way the partners worked. Her confidence in her achievement so far had been enhanced, and she felt encouraged to develop further.

The one-to-one nature of the appraisal interview, protected by privacy and confidentiality, allows people to be more open about their opinions, hopes and ambitions. This gives managers the potential for working out a better match between skills, aptitudes and tasks performed (George, 1991).

Example 6.4

A young practice secretary approached her appraisal interview with some trepidation because she knew that she had been making a lot of mistakes and had had a lot of sickness. She did not feel that she had much success to report, and felt depressed about her future.

The practice manager had noticed her depression and felt that it derived from a lack of job interest or prospects. She used the appraisal interview to check out the girl's skills and motivators. She found that she had been right in her assessment and that in addition the secretary found it very lonely in the practice office. She had actually always wanted a job working with people! She now found herself in a room on her own, generally with headphones on!

As a result of this formal interview, a training programme was planned to enable her to gain receptionist skills, and to stand in on a regular basis at the front desk. Targets and objectives were set to ensure an accurate record of achievement in her current job so that she was favourably viewed when a vacancy came up for a full-time receptionist. Further interviews were also set up to enable the practice manager to monitor the practice secretary's development.

Introducing an appraisal scheme

The steps involved in introducing an appraisal system are shown diagrammatically in Figure 6.2.

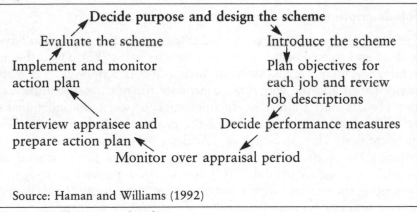

Source: Haman and Williams (1992)

Figure 6.2: The appraisal cycle

As with any management initiative, introducing an appraisal scheme into a practice will require careful thought and Box 6.3 summarizes the areas that need to be considered before doing so.

Box 6.3: Questions to ask before introducing an appraisal scheme
- What do I hope to achieve from the scheme – what will be its objectives?
- What form will it take?
- Who needs to be involved in its design?
- How can any objections, fears and anxieties about the scheme be best handled?
- Who will implement the scheme?
- What training will the appraisers and appraisees require?
- How much will the scheme cost to introduce and to implement?
- How should the scheme's effectiveness be evaluated?
- When should this evaluation take place?

Designing the scheme

Job descriptions

The introduction of an appraisal scheme requires the practice to have a clear and agreed sense of its purpose (Irvine, 1992). Once this is achieved it may be necessary to review job descriptions and staff performance and the way these contribute (or not!) to the organization's goals and objectives. Incongruities between an individual's activities and work objectives and the practice's objectives can then be identified. This updating of job descriptions is a good way of ensuring that staff are involved in the development of the scheme at as early a stage as possible. This is vital to a positive reception – presenting the practice with a *fait accompli* in the form of a designed scheme will not enhance its chances of success.

The job descriptions should describe what people do now and they are best created or updated in discussion with the job holder. Full details of how to write job descriptions are given in Chapter 1. However, it is important to be aware of the specific purpose of the job description in appraisal as listed in Box 6.4.

Box 6.4: Functions of a job description within the appraisal system

- It provides written information to the job holder of the requirements of the job.
- It is used to devise the method of assessment of performance.
- It provides the structure to help the appraisee and appraiser prepare for the appraisal interview.
- It provides the framework, for both parties, for the structure and content of the interview; it helps focus attention on work performance and avoids assessing character.

Methods of measuring and assessing performance

Measuring performance is usually one of the most difficult tasks to undertake in the design of a scheme, as much of the work performed in the practice relies on skills which do not lend themselves to quantifiable analysis. There is however a wide body of literature available to help in this, and the Industrial Society is a particularly useful source of information (*see* Appendix C).

Having said that, all managers will hold views on the performance of their staff, based on their observations and experience of working with the individual employees. One of the purposes of an appraisal scheme is to test the accuracy of these views, which may be based on patchy or inconsistent exposure to the work of the employees. This is particularly true for general practitioners. A lot of the humdrum work and the dramatic events encountered by receptionists go unseen by the doctor. Agreement on the ways to assess performance in these areas is vital in validating the assessment of the individual, and enables such 'hidden' work to be noted. The agreement could include consulting colleagues for their views of an individual, and ensuring that the appraisee has an opportunity to describe the full range of their job in writing or verbally.

Appraisal forms

Forms used in appraisal vary considerably, depending on the size of the organization, the purpose and objectives of the scheme, the level of the job being appraised and the method(s) selected to measure and evaluate performance. A popular format is for one form to be given to the appraisee and one to the appraiser to help each prepare for the interview. A third will provide a record of the appraisal interview including an action plan.

Details that need to be on each form are set out in Box 6.5.

Box 6.5: Contents of an appraisal form
- Basic personal details – name, position, length of time in the job etc.
- Terms of reference and a brief job description (or the job description can be appended to the form).
- Detailed review of the individual's performance.
- General comments including any extraordinary circumstances which have affected performance.
- Comments by the employee.
- An action plan including, if appropriate, any identified training and development needs.

The appraisee's preparation form should be designed to help the appraisee prepare for the interview. It could include the sort of questions set out in Box 6.6 which will encourage the member of staff to think about performance and future needs.

Box 6.6: Appraisal interview questions
- What have I done extremely well in work over the last year?
- What are the reasons?
- What have I done not so well?
- What are the reasons?
- What obstacles have I met?
- Do I have any skills/aptitudes which are not being used?
- In what areas do I need more experience and/or training?
- To help me in my job what action might be taken by: a) my manager, b) myself, c) the practice?

This preparation form is usually kept by the appraisee as an aide mémoire during the interview.

The appraiser's form is designed to ensure that considered thought has been given in advance to reviewing the employee's performance and thinking through strategies to help the appraisee improve. Above all, practices should endeavour to keep the paperwork simple, easy to understand and relevant.

Training

All staff involved in appraisal require training. Being appraised and conducting an appraisal interview are not easy tasks to undertake.

The interview – as in recruitment (*see* Chapter 1), in training (*see* Chapter 5) and in disciplining (*see* Chapter 7) – is a crucial part of the appraisal, and it is in dealing with this that many managers encounter serious difficulties which proper training can obviate. An appraisal interview is one of the most sophisticated interviews any manager can conduct. A badly handled interview can cause resentment, diminish staff morale and affect the credibility of the scheme. An interview which fudges sensitive or contentious issues will add nothing to the appraisee's performance. The appraisers – mostly managers or doctors – need to receive training in appraisal interviewing techniques, and appraisees need to be trained in preparing for the appraisal interview.

Resources needed

Time is the biggest resource needed to implement an effective system. Thus both parties need to be given adequate time, usually about a week, to prepare for the interview. For the interview itself, 30 minutes to an hour should be allowed for non-managerial staff and between one and two hours for the practice manager, the practice nurse or an associate principal.

The other resource is finance, as introducing and implementing an appraisal scheme is not cheap. Training is probably the most overt and easily calculated expense. In addition, the cost to the practice of the time spent on the design, implementation and continuous operation of the scheme should be assessed since this will be considerable when all the staff are involved.

Finally, it is easy to forget the cost of the materials involved in operating a scheme. Training materials may need to be costed in addition to the scheme's paperwork and photocopying or printing charges.

The appraisal interview

Much has been said already about what to do and not to do in interviews (*see* Chapter 1). However, unlike the recruitment interview, the appraisal interview is itself a development tool. The appraiser skilfully guides the appraisee to perceive and assess their own performance, and help them develop strategies to improve areas of performance which require attention. The appraiser must appear genuinely interested in, and committed to, realizing the appraisee's potential. Such confidence will occur if the appraiser uses the interview both to praise and recognize good work, and also to seek the appraisee's views on ways in which the appraiser can improve his or her management.

As with other management activities, appraisal interviews – if handled well – can reap enormous benefits. Handled badly, they have the potential to result in frustration, resentment and alienation. It is important, therefore, that everybody operating the scheme is trained in appraisal interviewing.

Preparation

As with all interviews, the quality of the preparation will largely determine the success of the interview. There are four major activities involved in preparing for an appraisal interview:

1 the collection and analysis of key information
2 devising strategies to improve performance
3 the interview plan
4 preparing the appraisee.

Collecting and analysing information

The appraisee's immediate manager is the most appropriate person to appraise the employee, being the most well informed about the appraisee and their current performance. Such knowledge is fundamental to the effectiveness of the interview.

Appraisal interviews should concentrate on performance and not personality, and should therefore be focused on the facts. It is important that views on performance from subjective sources, such as other colleagues or partners, should be tested against the facts.

Collecting and analysing information should not be left until the interview is imminent. Collecting information only a few weeks before is risky; it relies on memory and there is a tendency to concentrate on recent performance and to neglect past performance. It is important that appraisers have sufficient data to answer the questions set out in Box 6.7.

Box 6.7: Appraisal questions
- Has performance reached the standards expected in all, or only some, areas?
  - If so, what has contributed to this achievement?
  - If not, why not?

- Was the cause of failure the fault of the appraisee?
  - If so, what were the reasons?

- Was the cause of failure due to events outside the control of the appraisee?
  - If so, what are these and can they be influenced?

- What changes will be occurring in the practice which will affect the appraisee's job, and what are the implications for the appraisee?

CASE STUDY (11)

Cathy Colby, the new practice manager at John Street Health Centre, believed that one of her receptionists, Carol Field, was not really committed to her job. She was aware that this was a subjective feeling that needed analysis, and before the next appraisal interview she tried to analyse why she held this opinion, and to enumerate what aspects of the receptionist's behaviour led her to this view. The practice manager realized, after some thought, that her opinion was based on the receptionist's poor attendance record. There had been five periods of single self-certificated days sickness absence in the previous three months, and over the previous year the receptionist had refused every request to work overtime or to change her rota when other staff had been off work. By identifying the evidence which had helped form her opinion, the practice manager was able to test the accuracy of her belief, and she obtained the data to discuss it at the appraisal interview.

Cathy also used the preparation time to consider the strong points of the receptionist. Carol was most adept at handling the patients, particularly the awkward ones, and she was accurate and speedy in her clerical duties.

Cathy had now created a balanced context within which to conduct the appraisal interview, which was thus based on objective evidence rather than subjective feelings and emotions.

Devising strategies to improve performance

This is one of the most difficult areas to address in an appraisal interview as it is all too easy for the appraisee to become defensive or even aggressive. The preparation period therefore should not be confined to identifying objectively the areas to address, but also to think through (and even rehearse!) the approach the appraiser is going to adopt.

CASE STUDY (12)

Cathy Colby realized that there was little to be gained from labelling Carol's problem as one of attitude. She realized that her attention needed to be focused on the effects on the practice of the receptionist's behaviour. To do this she decided to start by discussing Carol's strengths with her first so that she was aware that her work was appreciated. Cathy then decided that a useful tactic would be to develop the discussion by asking Carol to analyse the tactics she used when dealing with difficult patients, with a view to using her experience and knowledge at an in-house training session. Building up Carol's confidence in her own abilities in this way would allow her to contribute to the performance of the practice as an organization. This could well increase her motivation at work.

Cathy hoped that at this stage in the appraisal interview Carol would be in a more receptive frame of mind to discuss her attendance record. The practice manager planned to raise this in a non-judgemental way and to focus on the facts, instead of opening the discussion saying: 'You have a very poor attendance record and it is causing the practice problems.' She realized that this would provoke a defensive response, where Carol would focus on justifying her absenses and nothing would be learned.

Cathy opted for a different tactic, saying: 'I want to discuss your recent bouts of ill health. You have had five periods of sickness over the last three months.'

This approach was non-judgemental and factual. Cathy hoped the discussion could then lead on to any problems she was having which could be the cause of the illnesses, and could be articulated within the context of 'How can I help you as your manager to improve your attendance record?' This could then be later followed by 'Are you aware of the impact on the practice when you are absent?' This line of discussion could then lead on to the notion of reciprocity – that other staff had to work longer hours or change their rotas when she was off – and help to discover how Carol thought her colleagues felt when she refused to do the same for them.

In the case study (12), Cathy planned to focus on behaviour and not personality. As it demonstrates, this strategy will not occur naturally. The appraiser needs to think through how topics are going to be raised, what the responses are likely to be, and how to develop the discussion constructively. It is helpful to write down the questions and openers that will be used during the interview.

Strategies which can consolidate and enhance current strengths need to be thought through. The example of actually getting a member of staff to assist in training others is one such strategy and is far more effective than merely saying 'well done'.

The interview plan

The outcome of collecting the information and devising strategies for improvement together form part of an interview plan. In addition the topics to raise, including training and developmental needs, should be listed, ensuring that the positives outweigh the negatives. As far as possible the negatives should be restricted to no more than two issues – more than that could make the appraisee feel intimidated or, even worse, that it is a disciplinary, and not an appraisal, interview. If the negatives do outweigh the positives heavily, then the manager should seriously think about how to deal with such a problem member of staff. It may be wiser to leave the setting of an appraisal interview until after a disciplinary or counselling interview (whichever is appropriate) has been conducted.

Preparing the appraisee

Appraisees must be given sufficient time to prepare, and it is helpful for them to be reminded of the purpose of the interview. Preparation forms can be made more specific by detailing the main areas of the employee's job and the skills required to perform the main responsibilities. For example, a receptionist's preparation form might contain the heading 'making appointments' and the receptionist is then asked on the form to assess their skills in communicating effectively. Equally it can include sections to enable the staff to comment on the manager's role in enabling them to do their job.

The interview

Even the most experienced appraisers feel some apprehension before an appraisal interview. Dealing with the unknown naturally produces stress and anxiety for both the appraiser and the appraisee. One of the purposes of the interview is to help the appraisee think through and discuss any difficulties, so the aim must firstly be to relax the appraisee.

The appraisee must be able to make full use of this opportunity to reflect objectively upon successes and failures both during and after the interview. The competence of the appraiser as a willing mentor is crucial in this process. Establishing rapport and allowing the appraisee to reflect on past performance can only be done if they have confidence in the integrity of the interviewer and are encouraged to talk. Chapter 1 sets out some strategies to help create a relaxed atmosphere in interviews (*see* Box 1.11).

Appraisal interviewing requires an awareness of the effect of one's own behaviour, particularly body language, and skilled questioning.

Non-verbal behaviour

People often pay far more attention to what they see than to what they hear. If body language and words are incongruent, it is the body language which is credited with giving the 'true' message. A person discussing an issue with clenched teeth is emitting signs of anger. It is the anger which becomes the focus of the recipient's response, rather than the actual issue under discussion.

Box 6.8 identifies key behavioural aids.

Box 6.8: Behavioural aids
- *Eye contact*. Establish and maintain eye contact throughout but do not stare or intimidate; ensure that the natural breaks taken to take notes are not prolonged.
- *Gestures*. Gestures reinforce but a repetitive gesture (eg pen tapping on a desk and finger pointing) can be aggressive.
- *Facial expression*. Have a relaxed, pleasant and smiling facial expression. Avoid serious frowning as this may be seen as disinterest or disapproval. Above all, do look as if you are listening.
- *Body posture*. Have a relaxed open posture indicating that

---

the interview is being taken seriously. This will encourage the appraisee to talk. However being over-casual – legs on desk! – will undermine the credibility of the interview.

Listening

It is very important to listen carefully as this is a rare forum in which staff can voice their opinions. New ideas and suggestions for developments often occur outside the planned agenda. Focused attention, with nodding to indicate agreement and the positive use of pauses will encourage the appraisee.

The body language of the appraisee may be important. If a suggestion is met with a verbal agreement but accompanied by a hesitancy in voice and body posture, it is a cue for the appraiser to probe more deeply.

Verbal communication

The interview should not be opened with a salvo of short questions. This may establish an interrogative mode which may be difficult subsequently to break. It is better to open with an easy question and to alternate questions of different types. Discovering both facts and feelings involves a combination of open and specific questions. The most valuable questions are those that start with 'what', 'why', 'how', 'where', 'tell me' and 'please describe'.

Box 6.9 sets out the type of questions that may be useful. More are given in Appendix A.

Box 6.9: Appraisal questions

Question	Example	Purpose
Open	'What areas of work do you think you've performed best over the last year?' or 'Tell me what you think of the new computer.'	To get the appraisee talking about ideas, feelings and facts.

Closed	'I understand from what you say that you aren't that keen on the new computer. Am I right?'	To summarize.
		To bring back to the subject at hand if the conversation has wandered.
		To check understanding.
Specific	'On average how much time each day do you spend on the computer?'	To find out the facts.
		Good for the verbose appraisee.
Reflective	You aren't entirely happy with the new arrangement?	Reverses a statement by rephrasing and sending it back to the appraisee.
		Keeps the appraisee talking.
		Avoids personal bias showing.
		Encourages the appraisee to expand the subject further.

Tackling problems

Appraisal interviews can be emotional minefields. Even so there is no excuse for not tackling areas of poor performance or fudging sensitive issues. Weaknesses are shared underlying problems; the question should be 'What can *we* do about this difficulty?'

Example 6.5
A receptionist was prone to abruptness with patients. The practice manager tackled this issue by saying: 'I want to talk about the role all our staff play in promoting the practice and this obviously involves our relations with patients. You are at the front line of this and play a very important part in the public relations of the practice. Have you ever thought of this part of your job?'
    The receptionist replied that she knew that being helpful was

very important. The practice manager then continued by
describing the following scenario:
  'Last Tuesday, Mr Fitzgibbon came in for his repeat
precription and you informed him that it was not ready, that
the practice needed at least 24 hours' notice and he should
remember this as he had just wasted himself a journey.
  Now tell me what you think of your reaction and put yourself
in the patient's shoes – how do you think he felt?'
  The interview then continued by discussing the receptionist's
own perceptions of her behaviour and her thoughts on the
patient's reaction.

In the above example, the appraiser has first placed the issue in context
and refrained from labelling the appraisee as rude or abrupt. The
incident was raised in a non-judgemental manner and the issue was
focused on the appraisee's behaviour and not her personality. After
all, there is little to be done about an individual's personality; changing
behaviour is the issue to address. Appraisers need to have the confidence to explain and justify their own behaviour – after all, the
manager may be the obstacle hindering the appraisee's performance!
Assertions must be clear, unambigious and supported by facts, not
feelings, and if issues are raised which cannot or should not be discussed, then the appraisee needs to be told clearly why such an issue
is off the agenda. If appraisee's become emotionally distressed, the
appraiser needs to keep calm and if necessary reschedule the interview.
  The case study (13) illustrates how, even with a poor start to an
interview, an appraiser trained in questioning and listening techniques
can use an appraisal interview to develop the appraisee effectively.

CASE STUDY (13)

Cathy Colby, the new practice manager, felt she was too new to carry out
appraisals of senior staff and so asked the senior partner, Bill String, to do it.
He agreed to attend a short appraisal course at the local polytechnic.

The senior receptionist, Betty Waters, had been with the practice for five
years, first as a receptionist and recently as senior receptionist. This was the
first time either Bill String or Betty Waters had undergone an appraisal interview;
they were both feeling rather anxious.

Dr String approached the interview from a position and briefing that indicated
that the practice was very pleased with Betty's performance – she was hard-

working, responsive to new ideas and seemed to get on well with the staff. She had a good relationship with the attached staff in the practice and patients. On occasions, however, she was slow to make and implement decisions especially if they might affect her popularity. She responded well to direction but rarely came up with any new ideas.

At 11.30 am Betty entered Dr String's consulting room for the appraisal interview. Her natural anxieties were balanced by the fact that she viewed herself as a conscientious employee who helped to keep the practice running smoothly. Nobody could accuse her of rocking the boat and she saw her position as carrying out the partners' instructions and keeping the new practice manager happy.

Dr String opened the interview by saying: 'Well Betty, let's get on with this and get it out of the way, shall we? It shouldn't take long. As I'm sure you know, Betty, the partners and Miss Colby are very pleased with the way you do your job. Tell me, what do you think you've done best over the last year?'

Betty was taken slightly off guard. She had been reading up on appraisals as Cathy had suggested and assumed that they would start by agreeing on the topics they would discuss. After a hesitant start, she replied: 'I get on well with everyone and the patients trust me. I think I work well under pressure and always make sure I get things done even if it means taking work home or working late. My enthusiasm for the new computer has had a good effect on the staff, even Joan Richardson who, as you know, was very reluctant to operate it.'

'Anything else?'

Betty continued: 'I can't think of anything else at the moment.'

Dr String referred Betty back to one of her initial points. 'Betty, you say you get on well with everyone?'

Betty: 'Yes.'
Dr String: 'Is that an important part of your job?'
Betty: 'Well of course. If I don't get on well with people, they won't co-operate.'
Dr String: 'What happens if you have to make or implement a decision that you know will be unpopular? How do you maintain good will?'
Betty: 'I usually manage to avoid making unpopular decisions. There's a way round these things, you know, especially now Cathy is here.'
Dr String: 'And what is your way round these things?'

(There was a long silence which was eventually broken by Bill.)

Dr String: 'Let's discuss some decisions which could have been unpopular: the computer, for instance. You say you helped to introduce the computer by your enthusiasm — what else did you do?'
Betty: 'I spent a lot of time telling the staff how we'd be more efficient if we had a repeat prescription system and the age/sex register on the computer. They seemed to agree and of course we staggered the training and introduced it gradually.'

Dr String: 'Good. I must say I thought the computer was going to be a real headache and we were all relieved when we realized that eventually the staff were as enthusiastic as the partners. Well done. Let's look at another decision – increasing the emergency surgery hours on Saturday? That decision was made three weeks ago. What's happened?'

Betty: 'Nothing.'

Dr String: 'Why is that?'

Betty: 'I just haven't had the time to discuss it with Cathy.'

Dr String: 'The time or the inclination?'

Betty: 'The inclination, I suppose. The staff won't like it and although I see the reason for it I know it won't be very popular.'

Dr String: 'Well, it has to be done, so how are you going to handle it?'

Betty: 'I really must take the bull by the horns and just tell them.'

Dr String: 'Do you think that's the best way of handling it?'

Betty: 'Why, what do you suggest?'

Dr String: 'I am not suggesting anything. But let's have a look at some other methods.'

Bill and Betty then proceeded to discuss ways of consulting the staff about the change of hours.

Betty: 'They still won't like it.'

Dr String: 'Or do you mean – they won't like you?'

Betty: 'Well yes. I won't be very popular.'

Dr String: 'Popularity is obviously very important to you. Do you think you won't be able to do your job if you are not popular?'

Betty: 'I have a problem which I want to raise with you. The staff still regard me as "one of the girls" and I find it actually impossible to exert my authority. I tend to pussyfoot around too much. Because of this, getting people to do things rests on how well liked I am.'

Dr String: 'Being promoted is always difficult, particularly when you now have to manage people who were your workmates. What can we do about it?'

Betty: 'I have given this some thought. I think I need my own office, like Cathy. Nothing elaborate. Just a private place where I can talk to staff in confidence. I also feel that the clerical and secretarial tasks I do for you undermine the supervisory role that Cathy keeps emphasizing.'

Dr String: 'That is a good start. I'll talk to Cathy about possibly creating some private space for you. I can't promise anything. If you can delegate some of the clerical and secretarial work to someone else then I assume Cathy will be happy. I hadn't realized its significance. If we do make these changes then I hope you too will change and find it less difficult to implement unpopular decisions. Betty, how do you feel about the partners when we make a decision you don't like. Do you suddenly dislike us?'

Betty:	'No. I don't agree with everything you do but I don't dislike you. I still respect you.'
Dr String:	'And that's the way the staff will view you. It's your overall style and the way a decision is introduced and implemented that affects the respect the staff have for you, not necessarily the decision itself.'
Betty:	'Yes. I see that now. It's not going to be easy.'
Dr String:	'Managing staff is never easy. It can be extremely difficult. I'd like to go back now and find out exactly what you are going to say to the staff about the new hours. . .'

After the interview

Shortly afterwards the appraiser needs to record the interview. The nature of this record is determined by the scheme's design. Whatever the design, the action plan and the identified training and developmental needs should be recorded. The record is then shown to the employee. Some schemes give a copy of the action plan and training needs to the appraisee.

If the scheme is to have credibility, it is important that the appraiser monitors and follows up any points arising from the appraisal interview and carries out any agreed action. Appraisal schemes which are confined to annual interviews without this ongoing activity degenerate into a paper exercise.

Evaluating the scheme

When a scheme has been firmly established it should be reviewed for effectiveness every three to five years, but when a scheme is first introduced, closer monitoring should take place. Large organizations can afford the luxury of a pilot scheme. Practices, due to their size, will find this more difficult. It is important therefore to assess a scheme's effectiveness fairly soon after it has been introduced and implemented. As with the design of the scheme, all participants need to be involved in this review process, and the areas to be covered are set out in Box 6.10.

The longer-term evaluation can only be conducted some months after the appraisal interviews have been completed. The degree of success of achieving the purpose of the scheme can only then be evaluated. However, many of the objectives of a scheme can be assessed during the immediate evaluation exercise.

Box 6.10: Review process
- *The training*
  - was it understandable, pitched at the right level and helpful in preparing and participating/operating the scheme?
- *The scheme*
  - was the preparation before the inteview helpful to the interview?
  - how long was spent on the preparation?
- *The interview*
  - assess the length of time taken to conduct the interview
  - assess the usefulness as an opportunity to exchange views
  - assess any change in the relationship between both parties
  - assess knowledge and insight gained

Conclusion

A commitment to appraisal involves far more than designing and implementing the scheme; it involves making value statements about its place in the overall organizational culture of the practice (Long, 1986).

Those value statements can be summed up as follows.

- Employees are one of the most valuable resources of the practice, who need to be cultivated, nurtured and cared for in a planned and considered fashion.
- High performance depends crucially on attending to people's developmental needs.
- Each person in the practice is entitled to have access to, and be able to discuss, information about their performance, skills and achievements, and to know how these are evaluated.
- Individual and practice performances are enhanced if information and knowledge are available, assessed objectively and skilfully discussed.

Box 6.11 sets out the prerequisites for a scheme to succeed.

Box 6.11: Prerequisites for a successful appraisal scheme
- The practice is clear as to the scheme's purpose and objectives.
- The scheme is vigorously supported by the doctors and the practice manager.
- Performance is assessed objectively.
- The design of the scheme is administratively convenient and fits into the culture of the practice.
- Its introduction is handled sensitively and involves genuine consultation with the staff.
- All involved in the scheme are adequately trained in the operation of the scheme and appraisal interviewing techniques.
- Action plans are implemented and monitored throughout the year.
- The scheme is regularly evaluated.

Performance appraisal is a valuable management tool in improving the individual and thus the practice – *if* it is done properly. Schemes which have not been skilfully designed and operated by trained managers result in a scheme which is at best of doubtful value, and at worst a minefield, abhorred and feared by appraisees and appraisers!

7 How to Discipline Staff

THERE are two elements in achieving and maintaining high standards. The previous chapter dealt with securing a general improvement for all staff through reviewing performance. The second element – handling the minority of cases of poor behaviour or performance through applying appropriate disciplinary procedures – is the subject of this chapter.

Why discipline?

The performance of any practice is eroded by poor standards of behaviour amongst members of the team. The purpose of a disciplinary procedure is to contribute to the maintenance of high standards and thus to help staff to improve.

However, there is a secondary purpose. Tolerating inadequate work or conduct gives the message to all staff that this is the accepted norm. There is nothing more demotivating for conscientious employees than for them to observe a colleague 'getting away with it'. Employees suffer frustration and stress when they feel obliged to compensate for the inadequate colleague through extra duties or through covering up shortcomings. Contrary to maintaining a caring image as an employer, avoiding addressing instances of poor conduct can cause dissatisfaction and unhappiness amongst staff.

The effect of low staff morale in a practice will also damage its reputation within the community as an enlightened employer. Ironically, it is the organization which delays addressing a disciplinary issue, and then eventually grasps the nettle, which in the end will be seen to have handled the problem badly. Over-hasty decisions taken in the heat of the moment, and warnings and dismissals which are eventually found to be legally unfair, all conspire to undermine staff confidence and respect and the practice's public image.

Consequently the financial and other costs incurred by practices who neglect their 'discipline' role can be enormous. Box 7.1 lists the most obvious.

Box 7.1: **Costs of neglecting discipline**
- High absenteeism.
- Staff working well below potential.
- Downright idleness.
- Falling patient lists.
- Recruitment and training costs either through staff turnover or a dismissal which could have been avoided had remedial action been taken at the right time.
- Industrial tribunal costs and compensation.

This chapter aims to give broad guidance on the law and practical advice to help deal with the variety of problems which fall under the 'discipline' umbrella.

Discipline and the law

Dealing with disciplinary issues is difficult for those general practitioners who see addressing such issues as conflicting with the profession's caring image. In addition, complications can arise if the member of staff concerned is also a patient of the practice. This attitude to discipline is compounded by the natural anxiety felt by many small organizations such as general practices at introducing a formal disciplinary procedure which may spoil the family atmosphere.

Many employers feel constrained by the complexity of employment law and erroneously believe that dismissing staff is almost impossible without risking industrial tribunal proceedings. It is undeniable that controlling conduct at work is affected by the rights and obligations imposed by law, but employment regulations and particularly codes of practice are designed to foster, not hinder, good relations between employer and employees. Far from preventing employers from taking disciplinary action, the law provides the framework within which disciplinary problems can be addressed. Most employment law relating to the termination of contracts of employment embodies what is good management practice.

The ACAS Code of Practice No 1 on Disciplinary Practice and Procedures in Employment (ACAS 1977) is the 'highway code' of industrial practice and provides the framework for all disciplinary codes. It is now supplemented by the ACAS advisory handbook *Disci-*

pline at Work which is intended to be 'user-friendly', and is available free of charge at any local ACAS office (ACAS 1987). Although not legally binding in itself, an employer who has to defend a claim for unfair dismissal in an industrial tribunal will be required to justify any breaches of the ACAS code's recommendations. It opens with the following helpful statement.

> 'Disciplinary rules and procedures are necessary for promoting fairness and order in the treatment of individuals and in the conduct of industrial relations. They also assist an organization to operate effectively. Rules set standards of conduct at work; procedure helps to ensure that the standards are adhered to and also provides a fair method of dealing with alleged failures to observe them.'

This statement is the key note of this chapter: it is the responsibility of practice managers and partners to ensure that the practice operates effectively and that their behaviour towards those practice staff who do not observe standards is consistent and fair.

The ACAS code contains a recommendation which must be regarded as a golden rule.

> 'An employee should be informed of any complaint against him/her and be given an opportunity to state his/her case before any decisions are reached. At all times the employer has a duty to behave reasonably both in the reason for a dismissal and in the operation of the procedure in arriving at that decision.'

All organizations which do have a disciplinary procedure are legally obliged to notify employees of their procedure. There is one exception – employees who commenced employment on or after 26 February 1990, with an employer who employs fewer than 20 staff, do not have this right to be given a copy of the rules. However the employer must still provide them with the identity of the person for whom redress of grievance may be sought. Indeed, it is good practice to ensure that, regardless of the number of staff employed, each employee is given a copy of the procedure.

Individual rights

Most employees have the basic right not to be unfairly dismissed. A duty to act fairly in dismissals is imposed on all employers by the Employment Protection (Consolidation) Act 1978. Box 7.2 lists the exceptions relevant to practice.

Box 7.2: Exceptions
Employees cannot take cases of unfair dismissal to a tribunal if they:

- have not completed two years' continuous service with their employer
- work less than 16 hours a week – unless they have been employed continuously by their employer for at least eight hours per week for at least five years
- have reached normal retirement age or are 65

However eligibility qualifications for bringing a claim for unfair dismissal, such as length of service with an employer, or age, do not apply to people who are dismissed because of sex or race discrimination, or because of trade union membership or activity. Protection against such unfair dismissal is obtained as soon as an employee joins an organization.

There are two riders to this. 'Continuous service' may include service with a previous employer, where for example a practice has been taken over. Secondly, if an employee who is close to the qualifying period of two years' service is dismissed without notice, then the statutory minimum notice period is included in calculating the 'effective' date of termination. For example, if an employee with 11 months' service is dismissed within one week of the second anniversary of the starting date, they will be eligible to claim unfair dismissal.

The law refers to five specific types of reason that may justify dismissal, as set out in Box 7.3.

Box 7.3: Justifications for dismissal
- Conduct.
- Capability (including health) or qualification.
- Redundancy – unless used improperly as an easier alternative to some other reason to effect a dismissal.
- If a statute would be contravened by continuing to employ.

- Some other substantial reason, eg:
  - difficult relationships with other staff
  - false information (which has importance) on an application form
  - reorganization of a business.

Fair dismissal

There are two factors in any dismissal which will determine whether it is fair or unfair.

1 Does the reason for the dismissal fit within one of the categories in Box 7.3 above?
2 Was the dismissal fair or unfair in all the circumstances having regard to equity or the substantial merits of the case? In other words:
  - has the employer acted reasonably in treating that reason as sufficient grounds for dismissing?
  - was the disciplinary procedure followed by the employer fair?

Industrial tribunals

Any claim for unfair dismissal by an employee must be lodged within three months of the dismissal although tribunals have discretion – very rarely used – to extend this time limit. To avoid a finding of unfair dismissal, an employer must demonstrate that the reasons for dismissing are related to one of the five reasons set out in Box 7.3 and – very importantly – that the employer acted reasonably and fairly when the dismissal took place.

To test this, the tribunal will be particularly interested in the organization's investigatory, disciplinary and appeals procedure, and whether the ACAS code of practice has been followed. It will also take into account the size and resources of the employer. A small organization is not expected to have as sophisticated procedures or the same resources to offer alternatives to dismissals (relocation, alternative work and so on) enjoyed by large organizations.

If an employee brings a claim for unfair dismissal the employer will have to spend time, resources and money fighting the claim. Staff morale may be affected and costly publicity damaging to the practice's public image and reputation may follow. It can also be an emotionally draining exercise, particularly for small organizations.

If the case is lost, compensation can be hefty. A tribunal award consists of:

1 a basic award equivalent to the redundancy benefit the employee would have received if they had been made redundant
2 a compensatory award which will take into account a wide variety of factors including how long the employee has been or is likely to be unemployed, and/or loss of wages and other employment benefits such as the loss of pension rights.

Financial compensation can be reduced if the tribunal assesses that the employee contributed to their own dismissal or has failed to mitigate any financial loss incurred as a result of the dismissal.

Also (although it is infrequent in practice) a tribunal can order a reinstatement or re-engagement with financial provisions against employers who refuse to comply. There are statutory maximum figures, adjusted annually on the amount of awards, but for the average practice these still represent substantial sums of money, particularly for long-serving staff.

Written reason for dismissal

After two years' service all employees have the right to be given the written reason(s) for their dismissal.

Notice periods

All staff have the right to be given notice, or pay in lieu of notice, on dismissal. The notice period must be the legal minimum – as determined by the length of service – or the notice specified in the contract of employment, whichever is the longer (*see* Chapter 2). Employees who are guilty of gross misconduct may forfeit any notice period or pay in lieu of notice, but the court or tribunal and the employer may not always agree on what is 'gross misconduct', and even in cases of the most apparent flagrant misbehaviour the disciplinary procedures should always be followed.

Handling a disciplinary issue

Before detailing the ACAS code, it is appropriate to repeat that the employer has a duty to act reasonably and fairly. It is an important part of all contracts of employment (*see* Chapter 2). All disciplinary interviews, from those for issuing a verbal warning to those which culminate in dismissal, should be characterized by reasonableness and respect for the employee. Staff will closely watch the manner in which a problem is handled and disciplinary issues which are managed hastily, inconsistently and with a loss of self-respect to the employee will lower staff morale in the practice.

The ACAS code highlights good management practice in disciplinary issues and the relevant section is précised in Box 7.4 with guidelines as to their application.

Box 7.4: ACAS code on disciplinary practice and procedures in employment

The disciplinary rules and procedures should:

- be written clearly and be available to all employees
- specify to whom they apply (if probationary staff are excluded from the full procedure, this should be stated)
- be designed to allow enough time for the disciplinary issue to be thoroughly investigated without taking so much time that the employee is caused undue stress
- indicate the disciplinary actions which may be taken, such as the obvious actions – verbal, written, final written warnings and dismissal – plus any alternatives to dismissal, eg suspension without pay or demotion
- specify the levels of management which have authority to take the various forms of disciplinary action and ensure that immediate superiors do not normally have the power to dismiss without reference to senior management. In general practice the practice manager usually has the authority to issue verbal (or even written) warnings to all ancillary staff but any decision to dismiss should only be taken by a partner. Allowing the practice manager authority to dismiss would be in contravention of this guideline
- provide for individuals to be informed of the complaints against them and to be given an opportunity to state their case before decisions are reached. The complaint(s) should be detailed in writing and followed by an interview. Enough time should elapse between receipt of the letter and the interview to allow the employee to marshal any evidence they may wish to present in defence
- give individuals the right to be accompanied by a trade union

representative or by a fellow employee of their choice
- ensure that, except for gross misconduct, no employee is dismissed for a first breach of discipline (examples of what constitutes gross misconduct should be specified in the rules)
- ensure that disciplinary action is not taken until the case has been carefully investigated, bearing in mind that comprehensive and detailed notes of the investigation may be crucial if a dismissal is referred to an industrial tribunal
- ensure that individuals are given an explanation for any penalty imposed verbally in a meeting and then confirmed in writing
- provide a right of appeal and specify the procedure to be followed informing the employee verbally and confirmed in writing; it is usual for the written warning letter or dismissal letter to explain the appeal procedure in the final paragraph

An example of a disciplinary procedure can be found in Appendix F.

Suspension

Occasionally the circumstances of a disciplinary case may make it necessary to suspend the employee whilst the complaint is being investigated. This option to suspend should be specified in the disciplinary procedure.

Any suspension should be on full pay and should be appropriate in length to the complexity of the complaint. Any dismissal following a suspension *without* pay, regardless of the fairness of the reason for dismissal, would probably be adjudged unfair by an industrial tribunal. Punishing a person twice (a period without pay *and* dismissal) for a breach of the rules is contrary to natural justice.

The disciplinary charge

If an employee is to be the subject of disciplinary action, they should be told of the particular complaint, followed by a letter containing the following:

- that the disciplinary procedure is being invoked
- the reasons why (the allegations should be specific and understandable)

- if appropriate, that the allegations are serious and *could* be grounds for dismissal
- documentary evidence, if appropriate, including copies of any previous warnings which relate to the disciplinary charge
- that the employee is requested to attend the disciplinary interview where a full opportunity will be given to answer the allegations
- the venue, date and time of the interview and an indication as to who will be in attendance
- encouragement to the employee to be accompanied; this not only demonstrates that you are behaving reasonably but also avoids any possible allegation of intimidation.

It is advisable to hand the letter personally to the employee. If this is not possible, send the letter by recorded delivery.

Figure 7.1 gives the disciplinary letter sent in the case study (14).

John Street Practice

Dear Julie

Further to our meeting this morning I am confirming that the practice's disciplinary procedure is being invoked and that you have been suspended from work, on full pay, for five days. You will be required to attend a disciplinary interview at 2.30 pm on Friday. The interview will be held in the practice manager's office, and I would urge you to exercise your right to be accompanied by a fellow employee of your choice.

As you are aware, the reason for this suspension is to allow the practice to undertake an investigation into the disciplinary charge which is that, unauthorized, you divulged confidential information about one of the practice's patients. This incident is alleged to have taken place yesterday evening at the Hope and Anchor public house at approximately 9.00 pm. The senior receptionist, Mrs Waters, has reported to me that she overheard you discussing with your boyfriend in a loud voice the details of one of our patients. I enclose a copy of her statement.

This disciplinary charge is serious and I must advise you that, under the practice's disciplinary rules, it may lead to your dismissal.

The disciplinary interview is your opportunity to answer the allegation and to present any evidence or mitigating circumstances of which you feel the interview panel should be made aware before reaching a decision.

The interview panel will consist of myself, the practice manager, and Dr Wood. Dr String will not be involved as he is the partner responsible for dealing with any disciplinary appeal.

When you commenced work with the practice you were given the practice's disciplinary rules and procedures. I now enclose a further copy.

If you are unable to attend the disciplinary interview please contact me or the practice manager immediately so that a mutually convenient time and date can be arranged.

Yours sincerely

Dr V Irons

Figure 7.1: Disciplinary letter referred to in the case study (14)

The disciplinary interview

Disciplinary interviews take place at various stages in the disciplinary procedure. They can take the form of either informal or formal meetings depending on the seriousness of the disciplinary charge. If the charge is serious and may lead to dismissal, the decision to deprive a person of their livelihood is not an easy one to take. Claims of unfair dismissal will often succeed or fail on the employer's conduct prior to and during the disciplinary interview.

The person conducting the interview should maintain an open mind. It should be viewed constructively, and thorough preparation – as with all the other interviews described in this book – is vital if a fair outcome, based on the facts, is to be achieved.

The enquiry

There are broadly two types of action to be considered when it is suspected or believed that an employee may have behaved unacceptably: an investigation and a disciplinary interview. Too often, employers move directly to the interview before all the facts have been investigated. First, therefore, everyone directly involved should be clear about the charge and what exactly is the reason for the interview. Then the employer needs to collect all relevant information, interview relevant witnesses and make notes of all pertinent facts. If after this exercise the employer is satisfied that some form of action needs to be taken, then the employee needs to be informed.

If the disciplinary charge is not serious, the interview can be informal and can be the opportunity to counsel staff in improvements to conduct or performance. It is important to be aware that an apparently trivial matter may be indicative of more serious underlying problems. Personal problems often manifest themselves at work in a deterioration in performance or relations with colleagues.

Verbal warnings should be recorded and the employee given a copy of the record which should contain the penalties for any further breaches. Warnings should have a life span (usually six months to a year) and this too should be specified.

Planning for the interview

As with all interviews – recruitment, appraisal, counselling – the disciplinary interview is best conducted in an atmosphere where, as far as possible, the employee can relax. The interview room should be comfortable and free of interruptions. If the interview is likely to be particularly stressful, arrange it for the late afternoon to allow the employee to go straight home afterwards.

Who should attend?

If the disciplinary procedure does not specify who should attend, there are three points to consider.

1 If possible, and particularly if the charge is serious, more than one manager should be in attendance. The ideal would be for one partner to chair, one partner/practice manager to present the facts and the other to take notes.
2 If the charge involves evidence from witnesses, these people should be in attendance. They should not, however, sit in on the whole interview. If a crucial witness is not able or willing to attend, a signed statement should be available and at hand to show to the employee.
3 The partner who will be responsible for hearing any appeal should not be in attendance. It is impossible to show that the principles of natural justice have been met if an appeal is heard by a partner who has participated in the disciplinary interview.

Box 7.5 sets out in summary form the pre-interview checklist.

Box 7.5: Pre-disciplinary interview checklist
- Are you aware of *exactly* what the complaint is?
- Have you obtained all the relevant data – dates, times, written statements, etc?
- Are you fully aware of the relevant facts and are they close to hand?
- Have you thoroughly investigated the complaint and anticipated likely explanations which may be offered?
- Have you made memory-prompting notes on the issues you intend to raise?
- Are there sufficient copies to hand of any previous warnings relevant to the case?
- Are you satisfied that those in attendance have been properly briefed, that witnesses have been contacted and that someone is responsible for taking notes?
- Is the room and the seating arrangement conducive to an undisturbed and, as far as possible, relaxed interview?

The conduct of the interview

Certain ground rules need to be observed in the conduct of the interview. The interview itself should follow a fair and systematic sequence. Its purpose is to ensure that all relevant facts and explanations are heard in order to establish whether disciplinary action is appropriate and the form it should take. It is *not* an interrogation, nor an opportunity for employers to vent their anger or displeasure on the employee.

The most satisfactory sequence is as follows.

1 The person chairing explains:

- how the interview will be conducted
- who will be present and why
- the purpose of the interview
- if the employee is accompanied, whether the companion is entitled to act either as the employee's representative or merely to provide moral support.

2 The complaint(s) against the employee is then clearly explained and the facts revealed by the investigation are detailed. If witnesses are to give evidence they are allowed to be questioned by the employee, and should then leave when each has finished.

3 The employee is then invited to respond generally and to call any witnesses on his or her behalf. These witnesses may in turn be questioned by the employer.

4 Any response to or further questioning arising from points raised by the employee should wait until the employee has been given a fair hearing without interruption.

5 Further discussions may be needed before all the facts are established. This discussion needs to be handled skilfully if it is not to degenerate into an unconstructive argument.

6 If new evidence is revealed during the course of the interview, further investigation may be needed. In this case the interview should be suspended and resumed once the second investigation has been completed.

7 At the end of the interview, the person chairing summarizes the main points raised by both sides.

8 The interview should then be adjourned to enable the interview panel to make a decision. There should be no pressure to reach a decision quickly. Depending on the complexity and seriousness of the case it may take a day or two to make a decision. The time taken, however, should not be so long as to cause undue stress to

the employee. Even in the most straightforward cases, the practice of adjourning – even if only for a few minutes – before making a decision is strongly recommended. It demonstrates that careful consideration is being given and it allows time to consider the type of disciplinary action to be taken. The options for action are set out in Box 7.6.

Box 7.6: Options for action
- A verbal recorded warning.
- A first or final written warning.
- Dismissing with notice or pay in lieu of notice.
- Summary dismissal (ie dismissal without notice or pay in lieu of notice) on grounds of gross misconduct.
- Demotion or suspension without pay (but only if this is specified as a permitted option under the contract of employment).

or alternatively

- Taking no further action on the grounds that the employee has given a satisfactory explanation of events.
- Taking no disciplinary action but arranging a counselling interview for the employee.

---

9 The interview may be reconvened for the employee to be told of the decision or notification may be given by letter. If the decision involves disciplinary action short of dismissal the employee should be clear about the matters set out in Box 7.7.

Box 7.7: Disciplinary action short of dismissal
Tell the employee about:
- the improvements that you require to be made
- any help the practice can offer, such as further training
- when you expect the improvements to be made
- any review period
- any penalties that may be incurred for further breaches
- the life span of the warning
- the right to appeal and the procedure to be used

CASE STUDY (14)

Julie Flower was the computer clerk/receptionist at John Street Health Centre. Julie had been with the practice for three years. Her work record was good and, although a little raucous at times, she was popular with her colleagues.

Betty Waters, the senior receptionist, reported to Cathy Colby, the practice manager, that the previous evening she had overheard Julie divulging confidential information about one of the practice's patients. This conversation was overheard in the local pub and the person Julie was talking to was her boyfriend.

Unauthorized divulgence of confidential information was a dismissible offence and this was clearly stated in the practice's disciplinary rules. In view of the seriousness of Betty's allegations Cathy consulted the partners. They agreed that a disciplinary interview should be held, and that Cathy should conduct it with Dr Veronica Irons.

Julie was informed in writing of the charge and that she might be dismissed (*see* Figure 7.1). She was given the date of the disciplinary interview and requested to attend on the due date. She arrived promptly at Cathy's office accompanied by her solicitor.

Dr Irons opened the interview by saying: 'Julie, you have received this letter detailing the alleged misconduct and that is why we are holding this interview. The purpose of this interview is to discuss the alleged incident so that we have all the facts before we make a decision as to whether the allegation is true and, if so, what disciplinary action to take, if any.'

Julie:	'This is a waste of time. You've already made up your minds. You've said so yourself in the letter – you are going to sack me. That's why I've brought a solicitor.'
Dr Irons:	'Dismissal was referred to in the letter because it's important for you to realize how seriously we view your alleged misconduct and to inform you that in accordance with the practice's disciplinary rules, dismissal may be an option open to us.'

Dr Irons then read out a statement that Betty had made.

Julie:	'It's just not true. Betty has never liked me and she's either made this up or she's mistaken. I *was* in the pub that night with my boyfriend but I didn't discuss any patient with him and I never would.'

Dr Irons then called in Betty who repeated her allegation. Betty was then questioned by Julie's representative. She denied disliking Julie and stuck to her story. She added that she felt compelled to report the incident not merely because it was a serious breach of the practice rules but because Julie was speaking in her usual loud voice in the pub and other people must have heard what she said.

Betty left the interview and Julie burst into tears. The interview was adjourned to allow Julie to compose herself and was reconvened some 10 minutes later.

Dr Irons:	'Now that you have calmed down, Julie, do you have anything else to say?'
Julie:	'What's the point? You have already decided whose story to believe, and even if I had said those things to my boyfriend, I'm not the only one here who does it. Don't tell me that you don't discuss your patients with your husbands and wives.'

Julie's representative then said: 'Julie has an exemplary work record. I believe she has never been disciplined before and if you do decide to dismiss, your evidence would be laughed at in court. To dismiss for a first breach of rules only on the word of one person would be unfair dismissal. I must inform you that if you decide to dismiss then I will be advising Julie to lodge a claim for unfair dismissal.'

Dr Irons: 'Julie do you have anything further to say?'
Julie: 'No.'

Dr Irons then closed the interview by telling Julie that she could now go home and that a decision would be made. She was asked to return to the practice at 11.00 am the following morning to hear the decision.

The practice decided to dismiss Julie. Their reason for dismissing was valid – misconduct. It was viewed as gross misconduct and was specified as such in the practice's disciplinary procedure. Although Julie did not admit to the misconduct the interview panel felt that they had sufficient evidence to sustain their belief in Julie's guilt; Betty was a long-serving and loyal member of staff and had no reason to lie, and although she had been anxious before and during her appearance at the disciplinary interview, she did not flinch when giving evidence.

Unexpected events

Disciplinary interviews are inevitably stressful events for all concerned, but particularly for the employee, and it is not uncommon for the employee to become distressed or argumentative. A short adjournment is often sufficient to allow the employee to compose themselves. Threatening behaviour or abusive language should not be tolerated. This type of behaviour should be treated as misconduct and the interview adjourned until a later date, when both the issue in hand and the subsequent misconduct can be dealt with.

A major difficulty arises when an employee refuses to respond during the interview. It is important to try to establish the reason why the employee is refusing to participate. If it involves a personal problem, the employer can offer the employee the opportunity to discuss the matter with the most appropriate partner or the practice manager. If this offer is rejected or if the refusal to respond does not involve a personal issue, the employee should be advised that such a refusal will mean that the panel cannot take into account any mitigating circumstances.

The disciplinary letter

With the exception of verbal warnings all disciplinary interviews resulting in disciplinary action should be followed by a letter stating:

- the reason(s) why the interview was held, and who attended. If the employee was not accompanied, it is advisable to include in the letter a statement such as: 'despite being aware of your right to be accompanied, you chose to attend the interview alone'
- what disciplinary action has been taken and detailing the consequences, if appropriate, of any further breaches of the disciplinary rules
- any improvements that are required, when they are to be made and any review period should be included, together with the right to appeal and the appeal procedure
- the notice period or pay in lieu of notice (if the decision to dismiss has been reached).

Figure 7.2 gives the disciplinary charge letter sent by John Street Practice in the case study (14).

John Street Health Centre

Dear Julie

Further to our meeting this morning, when you were informed of the decision of the disciplinary panel, I am now writing to confirm that decision.

As you are aware, a full investigation of the circumstances of the disciplinary charge against you has been undertaken. This included receiving evidence from Mrs Waters' alleging that you disclosed confidential information relating to one of the practice's patients. The details of the disciplinary charge were given to you in my letter of . . . .

Having considered all the evidence, including your comments at the disciplinary interview and those of your representative, it is with regret that I now write to confirm that the decision of the interview panel is to dismiss you with notice from your employment with the practice for reasons of gross misconduct.

You will receive three weeks' notice commencing on . . . .
and terminating on . . . . However, in order to give you
every opportunity to seek other employment you are not
required to work your notice period and you will therefore
receive three weeks' pay in lieu of notice.

You do of course have the right to appeal against this decision.
If you do decide to appeal, a letter stating your reasons for
appealing should be sent to Dr String within five working days
of receiving this letter.

Yours sincerely

Dr V Irons

Figure 7.2: Disciplinary charge letter

The appeal

The ACAS code recommends that an employee be given the right to
appeal. The appeal is the employee's opportunity either to restate
'their side of the story' or to present new evidence in their favour. On
receipt of notice of an appeal, the relevant partner who has not been
involved in the original decision needs to become familiar with all the
facts. If they are not satisfied with the thoroughness of the original
investigation, or the conduct of the disciplinary interview, or new
evidence is presented by the employee, a further investigation may be
needed.

After careful consideration, the employee and the members of the
disciplinary interview should then be informed of the decision. Informing the employee verbally and/or in writing will depend on the process
described in the practice's appeal procedure.

The decision will be *either:*

1 to uphold the original decision, *or*
2 to overrule the original decision.

If the decision is to overrule it then any lesser disciplinary action should be specified, eg a decision to issue a written warning may be reduced to a verbal warning. Again, the letter should follow the rules as detailed on page 125, although of course the right to appeal is not now applicable.

CASE STUDY (15)

Julie appealed to Bill String. Bill investigated the facts and felt that there had been insufficient investigation by Cathy and Veronica. If Julie had been divulging confidential information in such a loud voice, other witnesses should have been approached to strengthen Betty's allegation. Bill decided that this lack of investigation weakened the fairness of the dismissal. He consulted the practice solicitor and told his partners of his view.

He called Julie in to explain his decision to revoke the decision to dismiss, and to issue a final written warning instead. The decision left a legacy of bad feeling between Betty and Julie which was resolved some months later when Julie found herself a new position.

Forced resignation and constructive dismissal

There are two traps which can also lead to the doors of the industrial tribunal and of which all managers in general practice should be aware.

1 Forced resignation sometimes arises from what is seen as the easy option for losing an employee who is troublesome.

> **Example 7.1**
> A practice staff included a very rude and arrogant but long-serving receptionist, who was the wife of one of the local consultants and ex-secretary to the retired senior partner. The partners were sure that her behaviour was sufficiently obstructive and offensive to constitute serious misconduct but were loath to start full disciplinary proceedings against her, with all the aggravation that they saw would be involved. She was well aware of the practice's dissatisfaction with her performance, and had been heard to say that she expected 'to get her cards sooner or later'.
> Finally she was very offensive to a colleague in front of a

patient, and the partner with responsibility for staff took her aside and said: 'You are obviously aware that we are very unhappy about the way you behave and conduct yourself. You can hand in your resignation by tomorrow; otherwise the disciplinary procedure will be invoked and you will almost certainly be dismissed.'

The receptionist sent in her resignation, and the partners breathed a sign of relief. However, by the next post came news of her appeal to the industrial tribunal for forced resignation, and the awareness that the tribunal had the power to deal with this and treat it as a dismissal.

2 Constructive dismissal covers a multitude of potential employer errors. It describes the basis of an application to a tribunal by an employee who has not been expressly dismissed but who states that their employer acted in such a way that they were entitled to resign.

It can arise as a result of the employer committing a serious breach of contract, either of a specific term (such as a reduction of salary) or of an implied term (such as treating an employee in a way which destroys the relationship of trust and confidence which should exist between employee and employer). It may be that the employer acted in such a way hoping that the employee would leave, but this is not a necessary element in constructive dismissal.

Conclusion

It is impossible accurately to predict and anticipate human behaviour. It is far better for staff relations if disciplinary rules and procedures are firmly established before rather than after an event which may occasion disciplinary action. The very fact that there are no established rules and procedures may make any subsequent dismissal unfair. So far as the tribunal is concerned, if there is an established fair procedure, it will consider whether it was applied fairly. If there is no established procedure, the tribunal must decide (with hindsight) what the procedure should have been and then whether it was applied fairly.

It is also good management practice, regardless of the statutory requirements, to ensure that staff are fully aware of the rules relating to work, the penalties for breaching those rules and the procedure for handling breaches.

No matter how uncomfortable the partners and practice manager may feel in establishing written rules and procedures and adopting a more formal and detached approach when handing a disciplinary issue, it can be essential to the performance of the practice and in the prevention of tribunal proceedings.

8 How to Deal with Redundancy

THE issue of redundancy and/or redeployment is a very uncomfortable one, and does not sit happily with any of the previous chapters. However, it is an inescapable fact of modern life, and no book on managing people can avoid addressing it. First of all it is important to understand that one of the reasons for fair dismissal is terminating an employee's contract of employment for reasons of redundancy. The handling of a redundancy is prescribed in statute and current case law, in particular the Employment Protection (Consolidation) Act 1978 (EPCA). In addition to observing the law, any employer considering declaring an employee redundant also needs to be aware of, and sensitive to, the emotions surrounding a redundancy in the work place. A hasty, ill-considered approach can result in a level of uncertainty amongst staff which can adversely affect morale and performance.

Nevertheless, every organization's ability to succeed and change when necessary requires a review of how the staff are employed, and if the organization needs to restructure or shed jobs which have become obsolete, then redundancy may have to be considered.

The legal background

On the subject of redundancy, the EPCA states that:

'an employee who is dismissed shall be taken to be dismissed by reason of redundancy if the dismissal is attributable wholly or mainly to –

a) the fact that his employer has ceased, or intends to cease, to carry on the business for the purposes of which the employee was employed by him, or has ceased, or intends to cease, to carry on that business in the place where the employee was so employed, or

b) the fact that the requirements of that business for employees to carry out work of a particular kind in

the place where he was so employed, have ceased or
diminished or are expected to cease or diminish.'

In other words, when the work or type of work undertaken by
employees has ceased or diminished, a redundancy may occur. This
can include transferring work to another location or altering the type
of work undertaken in the organization.

Example 8.1
A part-time clerk had been employed to update the medical
records of a large seven-partner practice. The practice became
comprehensively computerized and each partner started to use
a terminal on their desk, allowing the medical records to be
updated by each doctor in the consulting room. Although the
work – updating medical records – had not ceased and the
location of the work had not been moved out of the practice,
the need for the part-time clerk to update records had ceased.
The part-time clerk's post was therefore declared redundant and
she was dismissed.

In the above example, the practice had a sound and logical reason for
changing the work of updating records from manual to computer
operation and in moving the work away from the reception area to
each doctor's consulting room. Had the practice merely decided to
alter the clerk's method of updating the records from manual to
computer and if this change had been within the clerk's capacity, then
any dismissal would probably have been found to be unfair.

It is not unusual for employers to try to use the label of redundancy
to dismiss staff they no longer wish to employ because they are not
satisfied or happy with their performance or conduct at work. Industrial tribunals are very aware of this practice and scrutinize such claims
of unfair dismissal thoroughly.

The issues to consider

There are several issues to consider when proposing to dismiss an
employee on grounds of redundancy, as set out in Box 8.1.

> **Box 8.1: The issues to consider when proposing to dismiss on grounds of redundancy**
> - Consultation.
> - Objective criteria for selection to be applied consistently.
> - Redundancy payments.
> - The alternatives to redundancy such as short-time working or work-sharing.
> - Inviting volunteers for redundancy.
> - Notice periods.
> - Alternative work.
> - Trial periods.
> - Time off with pay.

Consultation

Section 99 of the Employment Protection Act 1975 places an obligation on employers to consult recognized trade unions at the earliest opportunity. This means as soon as the employer proposes to dismiss employees. Although few practices deal with and/or have recognized agreements with trade unions, a House of Lords ruling in Polkey v AE Dayton Services Ltd (1987 IRLR 503) is relevant. That ruling stated that employers must consult individuals who may be dismissed. It is interpreted as meaning that, even where there is no recognized trade union, employers must consult those individuals they propose to declare redundant. In a more recent case (de Grasse v Stockwell Tools Ltd 11.11.1991 EAT 529/89) it was stated that whereas the small size of an organization may affect the nature or formality of the consultation process, it cannot excuse any lack of consultation whatsoever.

Such consultation must include putting the proposal in writing with the information outlined in Box 8.2. In the case of employees not covered by a union recognition agreement, the employer is not obliged to give a written statement of information, though it is still good practice to do so.

> **Box 8.2: Information which the employer must disclose**
> - The reasons for the proposals.
> - The number and descriptions of employees they propose to dismiss as redundant.

- The total number of employees, of that description, employed in the establishment.
- The proposed method of selecting the employees who may be dismissed.
- The proposed method of carrying out the dismissals including the period over which the dismissals will take effect.

Although there is no legal definition of consultation – other than providing the above information and considering and replying to any representations – case law has ruled that consultation must be meaningful and not a sham. The employer cannot go through the charade of listening to representations and then imposing a predetermined decision. This was made clear in the TGWU v Ledbury Preserves (1928) Ltd (No. 1) (1985 IRLR 412) where the Employer Appeal Tribunal (EAT) said that: 'There must be sufficient meaningful consultation before notices of dismissal are sent out. The consultation must not be a show exercise; there must be time for union representatives who are consulted to consider properly the proposals that are being put to them.'

Selection

The issues listed in Box 8.2 are not placed chronologically. Employers will often have some idea as to which employees are likely to be declared redundant before the consultation process begins. On the other hand part of the consultation process can include discussions on the method and criteria used in selecting staff for redundancy.

The system of 'last in first out' (LIFO) to select redundant staff is no longer the only way of selecting staff for redundancy. More sophisticated criteria for selection are being used by many organizations in order to ensure that a balanced workforce is maintained which can offer appropriate skills, flexiblity and adaptability. Whatever the criteria used, the method of selection must be reasonable and objective, and should be in accordance with any agreement or procedure/policy the organization has on selecting for redundancy.

Until fairly recently, redundancies in general practice have been rare, and few (if any) redundancy policies or procedures have been developed. However, if a practice decides that a redundancy situation is looming, it is good practice to develop a set of criteria which the practice can apply in selecting staff for redundancy. The earlier this is done the better. The selection criteria needs to strike a balance between consistency and flexibility and it is helpful to bear in mind that an industrial tribunal may well be in the position of scrutinizing these criteria for fairness and objectivity.

Example 8.2
Two practices in neighbouring areas decided to close or reduce their dispensing activities. In the first there was only one dispenser, so the dispenser's post was declared redundant. However, in the other practice the dispensary employed more than one dispenser and it was proposed to reduce the work of the dispensary rather than close it altogether. This practice had a redundancy policy which stated that three factors would be considered in selecting staff for redundancy: relevant qualifications, sickness record, and length of service. These were applied to select which of three employees was to be made redundant. One had been with the practice for 15 years, one had been there for three years, and one, the youngest, had been appointed two years beforehand. The employee with the longest length of service was the least qualified and had received counselling three months earlier on her poor sickness record. The practice decided to select her for redundancy using the above criteria. Her lack of relevant qualifications and poor sickness record outweighed the criteria of length of service.

The dismissal of an employee selected for redundancy is likely to be found to be unfair if the employee was selected for one of the reasons set out in Box 8.3.

Box 8.3: Unfair selection for redundancy
- The selection is in breach of a customary arrangement or agreed procedure, unless there are special reasons to justify the breach.
- The selection is for membership and/or activities associated with a trade union, or non-membership, or refusing to become a member of a trade union.
- The selection is discriminatory on grounds of race or sex, including women on grounds of pregnancy.

A claim for unfair dismissal may also arise if the employer has failed to undertake reasonable steps to offer employees alternative jobs within the organization. Industrial tribunals take into consideration the resources of the employer. A small general practice, for example, would not be expected to be able to offer alternative employment to the same degree (if at all) as a multinational organization.

Redundancy payments

Only those employees who have worked for the same employer for at least two years for 16 hours a week or more, or have worked for eight hours a week or more for at least five years, are legally entitled to a redundancy payment. Service before the age of 18 does not count. Employees who have reached the normal retirement age for their place of work, or are aged 65, are not eligible for a statutory redundancy payment regardless of the number of years service or hours worked per week.

The Department of Employment produces a booklet (DOE, 1990) with details of calculating redundancy payments. Statutory redundancy payment is determined by the employee's age, length of service and salary. Box 8.4 provides a guide to calculating these payments. When calculating a week's pay there is a statutory maximum limit of £205 per week (as at April 1992). The maximum limit is reviewed each year.

Box 8.4: Calculating redundancy payments
For each complete year of service, up to a maximum of 20 years, an employee is entitled to:
- half a week's pay for each year of service from age 18 and over but under 22
- one week's pay for each year of service from age 22 and over but under 41
- one and a half week's pay for each year of employment from age 41 and over but under retirement age

---

The redundancy payments described above are the payments employers are bound in law to provide for eligible staff. Employers can of course offer enhanced severance payments and indeed such enhancements can do much to alleviate some of the distress experienced by all concerned when members of staff lose their jobs through redundancy.

Notice periods

As with any dismissal, redundant employees are entitled to their contractual notice period or pay in lieu of notice. It is for the employer to decide whether or not they wish the employee to work all, some or none of the notice period. The circumstances of the redundancy may be such that it would be better for both the redundant employee and the organization if pay in lieu of notice is given. It also offers the leaver the opportunity to use the time to seek other employment. However, too much haste against the wishes of the employee (such as notifying the employee of the decision at 4.45 pm, stating that pay in lieu of notice will be given, and requiring that their desk be cleared by 5.00 pm) would invite sympathy from the tribunal, and might be seen as a defect in procedures or general fairness.

There are, however, advantages to the employee in working their notice period. If the employer is willing, the employee can use the facilities of the practice, such as secretarial services, for preparing CVs, or using the telephone to contact future employers. There is no legal requirement to offer these services, but it makes good sense to offer whatever help is possible and appropriate to the circumstances of each case. Not only is the practice helping the redundant employee to get back into the job market but it is also showing the rest of the staff that it is a considerate employer even when tough decisions have had to be made.

Alternative work

Even when the decision is made to declare a person's job redundant, the question of alternative employment is relevant to the reasonableness of the dismissal. Practices are small organizations, however, and it will be clear early on in the process whether or not there is suitable work for the employee to do. In Thomas & Betts Manufacturing Ltd v Harding (1980 IRLR 255), the Court of Appeal ruled that an employer should do what they can *so far as is reasonable* to seek to provide alternative work.

Where alternative work is found within the organization, the employee must be offered the new position before the notice period of the redundant post has expired. Where the new post is very similar to the redundant position in terms of the type of work and the terms and conditions of employment, any refusal by the employee to accept the offer could be viewed as unreasonable by the employer and the employer could refuse to make a redundancy payment.

Example 8.3

In a large nine-partner practice, one receptionist was assigned to each of the nine doctors to undertake clerical and some typing duties. Two of the partners decided to set up their own practice some 50 miles away. The practice had previously addressed the difficulties of working with such a large team, so the decision and consequent partnership break-up was amicable. The closure of the largest employer in the area, resulting in a migration from the area and a fall in the patient list, prompted the remaining partners to decide not to replace the doctors who were leaving.

On reviewing the work-load of the practice they decided that one of the full-time receptionist posts should be declared redundant. They selected purely on the 'last in, first out' principle. Sandra, the receptionist selected, was not unduly distressed. After four years at the practice she had become frustrated with working in such a pressurized environment and found her clerical duties boring. Notice was duly served. However, before the notice period expired, Sheila, another receptionist who was nearing retirement and had worked for the practice for over 20 years, requested voluntary redundancy. This meant that Sandra could be offered Sheila's post. The partners were relieved that no compulsory redundancy would have to take place.

However, Sandra refused the offer of Sheila's job. She could not or would not explain her reasons for refusing the offer. The offer was put in writing, the same duties and terms and conditions applied, and still she would not consider remaining.

After taking advice the partners decided that her refusal was unreasonable and informed her that if she did not accept the offer then she would not be entitled to a redundancy payment. She left and in law was regarded as having been dismissed by reasons of redundancy. Eventually the partners' decision to withhold a redundancy payment was upheld.

In Example 8.3 the employee left even though she forfeited her redundancy payment. Employers have to weigh up the advantages and pitfalls of exercising this right not to make a redundancy payment where an offer of suitable employment is refused. A situation can arise where the employee agrees reluctantly to accept the offer. Employing disgruntled staff who are not working for the practice through choice can be more expensive in the long term than making a redundancy payment. The disaffection felt by the member of staff can affect their performance at work and the morale of the surgery.

Trial periods

Where the alternative work offered differs from the redundant position, the employee has the right to try it out. Where the new job is different in the type of work, the status, location, hours of work or any other significant terms and conditions of employment, then the redundant employee must be allowed a trial period of four weeks (or longer if the employer agrees) to decide whether the new job is suitable without necessarily losing the right to a redundancy payment. The employer too can use the trial period to assess whether or not the employee is suitable for the new job. Should the employee leave during the trial period because the new post is not suitable, or should the employer dismiss the employee due to their unsuitability, the employee does not forfeit the right to a redundancy payment and is treated as if the redundancy took place at the expiration of the original notice period. However, if the employer does dismiss during the trial period for a reason unconnected with redundancy, for example gross misconduct, then the employee may lose the redundancy entitlement. In such a case, the employer may have to justify the dismissal in the normal way before a tribunal and all the usual disciplinary procedures should be applied in the normal way.

Alternative offers of employment, and particularly those which attract a trial period, should be detailed in writing, stating the date when the trial period starts and finishes, and the measures which will be used to assess the employee's suitability. All offers of alternative work must be made before the employee's contractual notice period has expired and taken up either immediately after the end of the old job or after an interval of not more than four weeks.

Time off with pay

Employees who are under formal notice of redundancy have the right to reasonable time off with pay, in working hours, to look for work or to make arrangements for training for future employment. A tribunal can make a financial award against the employer if they unreasonably refuse this right to employees under notice of redundancy. Employees with less than two years' service, or less than five years' service if they work for between eight and 16 hours per week, are not eligible for this right. However it is good management practice, regardless of the hours worked or the years of service, to allow staff paid time off to make such plans for their future.

Managing redundancy

The practice which decides to embark on a redundancy needs to think through very carefully not only the legalities of the process but also the emotional and practical needs of the employee, and the effects on the staff who are staying and the people in the practice who are actually handling the redundancy. In all the issues described above, reference has been made to the value of looking beyond the legal requirement at each stage.

If the practice handles a redundancy insensitively it is remembered by those who stay as well as those who are being made redundant. Trust and confidence can be more easily damaged by a badly handled redundancy than almost any other single event in an organization.

Once the process of consultation and selection has been undertaken, the communication of the decision should be given the highest priority in the management of the practice at that time.

Breaking the news

Obviously the staff selected need to be informed first. The meeting where the proposal to select the person is communicated should be very short, as most people, when given news of this nature, cease to hear anything after that.

Counselling

Even before the final decision is made and during the consultation process, employees may have feelings of anger and even bereavement which need to be explored and dealt with before a constructive attitude to opportunities for new work can be adopted. The practice should not be tempted to undertake this counselling role in house. If a member of staff is experiencing these emotions, even if counselling is a speciality of the practice, the practice must retain the detached employer role. A reputable 'outplacement' company can do much to help redundant staff, or of course the employee can be referred to a variety of professionals who can offer counselling.

Practical help

The distress of redundancy cannot be over-emphasized, and most people need reassurance in their worth as employees and practical help in seeking new employment. Frequently the employee does not realize that the decision to dismiss was difficult and that it does not reflect on their value as a person. Reassurance needs to be made verbally explicit and sincere expressions of regret should be included in the letter of termination of employment. Providing open references, contacting other practices who may have vacancies, and providing resources and assistance to the employee, will help alleviate some of the more immediate stresses on the individual and on the practice.

The staff and colleagues who remain may go through a period of guilt and grieving; unsure of their own futures in the practice, they too need to be given reassurance. Handling a redundancy professionally, sympathetically and generously (both in money and the time the key players can spend in planning and managing the redundancy) can do much to maintain the morale of the staff and the partners of the practice.

Conclusion

Although redundancy no longer carries the stigma it once did, the act of depriving a person of their employment should never be taken lightly. It can be a very distressing experience, and redundancies which take place during an economic recession, where opportunities to gain new employment are limited, can be traumatic.

A person's sense of self-respect and worth is often tied up with the work they do. A fall in income is only one of the most obvious effects of redundancy; the emotional and psychological impact of such a dismissal can be profound. Ensuring that the practice complies with the statutory requirements, and handles redundancies with sensitivity and confidence, will enable the organization to address and manage effectively one of the most difficult issues facing organizations in contemporary British society. It will also reflect the sophistication and professionalism of the practice's approach to, and knowledge of, the most sensitive and effective ways of caring for its staff as well as its patients.

Appendix A: Questioning Techniques

Closed questions usually call for a straight 'yes' or 'no' answer. As such their usefulness is limited, but they are useful in checking levels of existing knowledge, particularly in training sessions.

Open-ended questions are much more useful. They are aimed at producing answers as a series of facts or expressions of opinion.

  i) factual questions, eg 'What are the purposes of medical audit?' call for a definite answer and are very useful. They require the other person to think and consider before answering. The interviewee is not led into giving an answer.

  ii) general questions, eg 'Why did you apply for this post?' allow the interviewee to select the information and allow the interviewer to identify the interviewee's priorities, areas of interest, and powers of articulation.

Multiple questions give choice, eg 'Would you rather make people attend training courses or motivate them to attend voluntarily?' They lead the person into considering only the choices you have posed in the question. People will often choose the alternative they think you want to hear.

Leading questions indicate the answer the questioner wants, eg 'You are not going to do it that way are you?' Unless the questioner deliberately wants to provoke, there is very little to recommend this type of question.

Overhead questions call for an explanation, eg 'What do we mean by the term good practice?' This question is useful in helping to get a discussion group to contribute to a training session.

Controversial questions introduce an element of provocation, eg 'Has
the 1990 contract made life easier for practice staff?'

Redirected questions maintain participation, eg 'Jenny here has asked
whether we should bring in outside consultants. What
do you think?' This is particularly useful when running
discussion groups.

Appendix B: Relevant Legislation

Access to Medical Records Act 1988
Congenital Disabilities (Civil Liability) Act 1976
Data Protection Act 1984
Disabled Persons (Employment) Acts 1944 & 1958
Employment Acts 1980, 1982, 1989
Employment Protection Act 1975
Employment Protection (Consolidation) Act 1978 (EPCA)
Equal Pay Act 1970
Equal Pay (Amendment) Regulations 1983
Health and Safety at Work Act 1974
Race Relations Act 1976
Rehabilitation of Offenders Act 1974 and Exceptions Order 1979
Sex Discrimination Act 1975
Social Security Act 1986
Trade Union and Labour Relations (Consolidation) Act (TULR [C]A)
Trade Union Reform and Employment Rights Bill 1992
Unfair Contracts Terms Act 1977
Wages Act 1986

Appendix C: Useful Addresses

1. Institute of Personnel Management
   PM House, Camp Road, London
   SW19 4UX   Tel.: 081–946 9100

2. Data Protection Registrar,
   Springfield House, Water Lane,
   Wilmslow, Cheshire SK9 5AV   Tel.: 0625 535777

3. Health and Safety Committee,
   Baynards House, 1 Chepstow Place,
   Westbourne Grove, London W2 4TF   Tel.: 071–221 0870

4. Advisory, Conciliation and Arbitration
   Service (ACAS),
   Head Office: 27 Wilton Street, London
   SW1X 7A   Tel.: 071–210 3000

5. Whitley Councils for the Health
   Services (Great Britain)
   Quarry House
   Quarry Hill
   Leeds LS2 7HU   Tel.: 0532 545000

6. Association of Health Centre and
   Practice Administrators (AHCPA),
   c/o 14 Princes Gate, London SW7 1PU   Tel.: 071–581 3232

7. Association of Medical Secretaries and
   Practice Administrative Staff
   (AMSPAR),
   Tavistock House North, Tavistock
   Square, London WC1H 9JR   Tel.: 071–387 6005

8. Royal College of General Practitioners
   (RCGP),   Tel.: 071–581 3232
   14 Princes Gate, London SW7 1PU   Fax: 071–225 3046

9. British Medical Association (BMA),
   Tavistock Square, London WC1H 9JR   Tel.: 071–387 4499

10. Royal College of Nursing (RCN),
    20 Cavendish Square, London W1M
    9AE   Tel.: 071–409 3333

11. The Industrial Society,
    Peter Runge House, 3 Carlton House
    Terrace, London SW1Y 5DG   Tel.: 071–839 4300

Appendix D: Individual Rights Arising From Employment

THIS list is not exhaustive but it does cover the major statutory employment rights of employees. There are exceptions to eligibility to many of these rights which are not appropriate to list here. This list is a general guide only.

Many rights are determined by hours of work and length of service. Where there are no such qualifying factors (ie all employees have the entitlement), the individual right is marked +.

	Individual right	Legislation
	Time off work	
	for public duties	Employment Protection (Consolidation) Act 1978
	to seek alternative work or to arrange training in a redundancy situation	Employment Protection (Consolidation) Act 1978
+	to receive antenatal care	Employment Act 1980
	to carry out trade union duties or IR training, if trade union is recognized for collective bargaining purposes	Trade Union and Labour Relations (Consolidation) Act 1992
	to carry out trade union activities if the trade union is recognized	
	Time off with pay	

Access to information

+ to have access to personal data held on employer's computer — Data Protection Act 1984

+ to have access to medical reports provided by a medical practitioner for employment purposes — Access to Medical Reports Act 1988

Wages and salaries

+ to receive equal pay and terms and conditions with a member of the opposite sex doing work rated as equivalent or of equal value — Equal Pay Act 1970 and Equal Pay (Amendment) Regulations 1983

+ not to have deductions made from salaries unless contractually agreed or required by statute — Wages Act 1986

to receive an itemized pay statement — Employment Protection (Consolidation) Act 1978

to receive a guaranteed payment when no work is available — Employment Protection (Consolidation) Act 1978

to receive statutory sick pay — Social Security and Housing Benefit Act 1982

*Maternity**

to receive statutory
   maternity pay

Social Security Act 1986
Employment Protection
(Consolidation) Act 1978
and Trade Union Reform and
Employment Rights Bill
1992

to return to work after
   absence on maternity
   leave

Employment Act 1980 and
Social Security Act 1986

+ not to be dismissed on
   grounds of pregnancy

Sex Discrimination Act 1975

* At the time of writing the Trade Union and Employment Rights Bill is in
Committee stage of its passage through Parliament. If the proposals in the
Bill are adopted and passed as law, then maternity provisions, both leave
and pay, will be affected.

Discrimination

+ not to suffer discrimination
   on grounds of sex,
   marital status, colour,
   race or nationality in
   terms of recruitment and
   selection, training,
   promotion, dismissal

Sex Discrimination Act 1975
and Race Discrimination
Act 1976

+ to conceal past convictions
   where the conviction
   has become spent

Rehabilitation of Offenders
Act 1974

+ not to have action, short of
   dismissal, taken against
   oneself because of trade
   union membership or
   activity

Trade Union and Labour
Relations (Consolidation)
Act 1992 and Employment
Protection (Consolidation)
Act 1978

Written terms of
*employment**

+ to receive a written   Employment Protection
    statement of the main   (Consolidation) Act 1978,
    terms and condition of   Trade Union Reform and
    employment within 13   Employment Rights Bill 1992
    weeks of commencing
    employment (employees
    who work eight hours a
    week or more but less
    than 16, within 5 years)

* At the time of writing the Trade Union and Employment Rights Bill is in
Committee stage of its passage through Parliament. If the proposals in the
Bill are adopted and passed as law, then the format and timing of written
terms of employment will be affected.

Termination
to receive a minimum   Employment Protection Act
    period of notice based   1975
    on length of service
    (after four weeks' service)

to receive a redundancy   Employment Protection
    payment   (Consolidation) Act 1978

in a redundancy situation,   Employment Protection Act
    to be entitled to a trial   1975
    period, where alternative
    employment is offered,
    without forfeiting right
    to redundancy payment

to receive a written   Employment Protection
    statement of the reasons   (Consolidation) Act 1978
    for dismissal

	not to be unfairly dismissed	Employment Protection (Consolidation) Act 1978 and Employment Act 1980
+	on the grounds of: sex and marital status (including pregnancy)	Sex Discrimination Act 1975
+	race, colour or nationality	Race Relations Act 1976
+	trade union membership or activity	Trade Union and Labour Relations (Consolidation) Act 1992

Appendix E: Training Techniques

Role-play   In the training session, trainees enact the role they will be called upon to play in their work. This is usually used to practise face-to-face situations; interviewing skills training often uses this method.

Uses   The trainee can practise a near-life scenario and receive expert advice and comments from their peers in a 'protected' environment. It gives confidence and the trainee gets the feel of a real-life situation.

Pitfalls   Trainees may feel self-conscious and, unless handled well, trainees can lose confidence. It can also be viewed as a 'bit of a lark' and not taken seriously.

Case study   The trainees – in groups or individually – examine the history of an event or set of circumstances. There are two categories: the trainee diagnoses the cause of a particular problem, and the trainee sets out to solve a particular problem.

Uses   This is suitable where a cool look at the problem, free from the pressures of the actual event, is beneficial. It provides opportunities to exchange ideas and to consider possible solutions to a problem the trainee will face in work.

Pitfalls   Trainees may get the wrong impression of what happens in reality. They may fail to appreciate that decisions taken in the training exercise will differ from those taken on the spot in the work environment.

Lecture   A talk is given without any participation from the audience.

Uses   It is suitable for large audiences where participation is not possible because of the numbers. It is a technique used to give information.

Pitfalls   The lack of participation means that, unless the whole of it is understood from beginning to end, the sense will be lost.

Talk   A talk is designed to encourage participation. It may use a variety of techniques, and participation is usually in the form of questions.

Uses   It is suitable for putting across information to groups of no more than about 30 people. Participation maintains interest and helps the learning process.

Pitfalls   If trainees do not want to participate, the talk will turn into a lecture.

Discussion groups   Knowledge, ideas and opinions on a particular subject are freely exchanged among trainees and discussion leader.

Uses   It is suitable for solving problems or inducing/changing attitudes. It is also a means of obtaining feedback on the way trainees may apply the knowledge learned.

Pitfalls   Trainees have to be skilfully but unobtrusively managed if the discussion is to involve all. It is important to prevent domination by one person and to ensure that discussion does not stray or become entrenched.

Job instruction   A trainee is told or shown how to do a job/task, or the trainee does the job/task under supervision (talk, demonstration or practice)

Uses   It is suitable for skills training. The job is broken down into 'learnable chunks' which are practised. The whole skill is thus built up in easily understood stages, which gives the trainee confidence.

Pitfalls	Thorough, clear instruction involving comprehensive preparation is vital. The trainee needs to feel relaxed about making mistakes.
Exercises	Trainees are asked to perform a particular task leading to a required result. Trainees use the exercise to put into practice information/knowledge they have been given. Exercises may also be used to assess trainees' existing knowledge before training begins/recommences.
Uses	Exercises can be used for groups or individual work, where trainees need to practise a particular skill or formula in order to achieve an objective. This is a highly active technique and has a lot of scope for the imaginative trainer.
Pitfalls	The exercise must be realistic and the expected result achievable; otherwise trainees will lose confidence or feel frustrated.
Project	This is similar to an exercise but gives the trainee a lot of scope to develop and demonstrate creativity and initiative. A particular task is given but the methods – or even the actual topic – are for the trainee to determine. Projects can be set for groups or individuals.
Uses	A project may be suitable where initiative and creativity need developing. It can provide feedback on a range of personal qualities as well as knowledge and attitude, and give a lot of scope for the imaginative trainer.
Pitfalls	Trainees must be interested and co-operative. The topic must be relevant to their needs. A failure will have a far more dramatic impact on the trainee than a failure in any of the other methods.

Appendix F: Sample Disciplinary Procedure

THE practice expects all staff to observe and maintain satisfactory standards of performance and behaviour. This procedure has been prepared to help employees meet these standards. The practice, as the employer, will advise, counsel and train staff. These are not in themselves disciplinary functions unless they are related to unsatisfactory behaviour as described below.

Minor breaches of rules

Failure to meet performance standards, minor misconduct (eg poor time-keeping and minor infringements of the practice's health and safety at work policy) will result in an informal meeting with the practice manager where a verbal warning may be issued. A record of the meeting will be given to the employee.

It is expected that in most cases a verbal warning will quickly resolve most difficulties. Where there is a more serious case of misconduct or an employee fails to improve and maintain that improvement with regard to conduct or job performance, the case will be treated as a serious breach of rules.

Serious breach of rules

While the following list is not exhaustive, this may be taken to include:

  i repetition of breaches of discipline which have occasioned a previous warning
 ii insubordination
iii wilful or serious breach of the practice's health and safety at work policy
 iv unauthorized removal of the practice's property
  v any illegal act of discrimination on the grounds of sex or race

   vi neglect of duties or refusal to carry out reasonable instructions
   vii flagrant failure to follow documentary procedures and regulations
  viii working for another employer without the prior express agreement of the practice
   ix behaviour outside work which is likely to have an adverse effect on the practice's reputation or if the behaviour makes the employee unsuitable to hold their position
   x breaches of confidentiality.

The circumstances of the event will be reported by the practice manager to Dr . . . . . . who will conduct an enquiry and make the necessary investigations. If as a result of the enquiry a disciplinary interview is convened the employee will be:

   i given the right to be accompanied by a fellow employee
   ii informed of the nature of the complaint and such evidence as may exist
  iii given the opportunity to present their explanation of the matter, including any mitigating circumstances.

If it is decided that disciplinary action should be taken, the employee will be told of the decision and later given a letter confirming:

   i details of the complaint that has occasioned the written warning
   ii the necessary action to remedy the situation, any period of review, extra training etc decided upon
  iii that any further repetition or instances of misconduct (as appropriate) will result in:
     – a further disciplinary interview which may result in a final written warning, which if unheeded may result in dismissal with appropriate notice, *or*
     – dismissal with appropriate notice
   iv the employee's right to appeal and the appeal procedure.

The final decision to dismiss can only be taken by Dr . . . . , or in their absence Dr . . . . , after they have conducted a thorough investigation into the circumstances of the case, are satisfied with regard to the facts of the case and the appropriateness of any mitigating circumstances and after interviewing the employee.
   Alternatives short of dismissal may be considered. They are:

   i suspension without pay up to a maximum of seven days
   ii demotion or transfer to another job, if available.

Summary dismissal

In rare circumstances the employee may be summarily dismissed without notice, if it is established – after investigation and after hearing the employee's version of the matter – that there has been an act of gross misconduct. In cases of gross misconduct, the practice reserves the right to dismiss without notice.

The following list is not exhaustive but such acts include:

   i theft
  ii fraud
 iii abuse of drugs
  iv being under the influence of drink and drugs during working hours
   v wilful unauthorized disclosure of confidential information
  vi unauthorized removal of any patient or administrative records from the practice
 vii deliberate damage to practice property or that of other employees
viii disorderly or indecent conduct, fighting on practice premises or threatening physical violence
  ix acts of incitement or wilful acts of discrimination on the grounds of sex or race.

Generally in connection with disciplinary procedures

1 At any disciplinary interview or meeting at any stage in the disciplinary procedure, the employee will be given details of the complaint or allegation, will be given full opportunity to explain or defend themselves and have the right to be accompanied by a fellow employee.
2 In certain circumstances, the practice may suspend an employee from duty whilst the circumstances of the disciplinary charge are being investigated. Any such suspension will be on full pay.
3 A copy of any written warning, or record of a verbal warning, will be retained on file. The length of time the warning will remain effective will be determined by the circumstances of the case. Only in exceptional circumstances will a warning remain effective for more than one year. The employee will be informed of the length of time applicable to any specific warning.
4 The employee may appeal against any disciplinary action taken

against them. The appeal should be made in writing to Dr . . . .
unless they have been involved in the disciplinary decision, then the
appeal should be made to Dr . . . . Any such appeal should
be made within five working days of receipt of the warning or
dismissal.

Practice manager

The practice's disciplinary procedure applies to the practice manager.
However, the authority to conduct a disciplinary enquiry, interview,
warning or dismissal can only be taken by Drs . . . . and . . . .

Probationary staff

The full disciplinary procedure is not intended to apply to a member of
staff during their probationary period, during which time any measures
taken and procedures adopted shall be wholly at the discretion of the
partners.

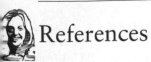

References

ACAS (1985) *Code of practice for the elimination of racial discrimination and the promotion of equality of opportunity in employment.* HMSO, London.

ACAS (1977) *Code of practice on disciplinary practice and procedures in employment.* HMSO, London.

ACAS (1987) *Discipline at work.* HMSO, London.

ACAS (1985) *Code of practice for the elimination of discrimination on the grounds of sex or marriage, and the promotion of equality of opportunity of employment.* HMSO, London.

DOE (1990) *Redundancy payments.* HMSO, London.

Drury M (1990) (Ed) *The new practice manager.* Radcliffe Medical Press, Oxford.

Ellis N (1990) *Employing staff.* British Medical Journal, London.

Ellis N (1992) The GP as employer – are you responsible? *Management in General Practice.* **4**, 46–4.

Fowler A (1991) How to conduct interviews effectively. *Personnel Management Plus Magazine.* **2**, No. 6

George J (1986) Appraisal in the public sector: dispensing with the big stick. *Personnel Management.* **5**: 32–5.

Haman H and Williams S (1992) *Putting appraisal into practice.* Department of Postgraduate Studies, UWCM, Cardiff.

Hancy C (1991) *The age of unreason.* Business Books, London.

Harvey-Jones J (1988) *Making it happen.* Fontana/Collins, London.

Hogg, C (1988) (Ed) *Fact sheet 3.* Personnel Management (3).

Hunt J (1990) *Managing people at work* (2nd ed.). McGraw Hill, London.

Irvine D and Irvine S (Eds) (1991) *Making sense of audit.* Radcliffe Medical Press, Oxford.

Irvine S and Huntington J (1991) *Management appreciation – the book.* RCGP, London.

Irvine S (1992) *Balancing dreams and discipline.* RCGP, London.

Long P (1986) Performance appraisal revisited. IPM *Personnel Management Plus* 1990, London.

Melton K and Long M (1990) Delegation: how to spread the load. *Modern Medicine*. 35, 409–10.

Plant R (1987) *Managing change and making it stick*. Fontana/Collins, London.

Prentice G (1990) Adapting management style for the organisation of the future. *Personnel management*. 6, 58–62.

Pringle M *et al.* (1991) *Managing change in primary care*. Radcliffe Medical Press, Oxford.

Royal College of General Practitioners (1985) *Management in practice*. Video and course book. RCGP, London.

Royal College of General Practitioners (1986) *We need a practice manager*. Video and course book. RCGP, London.

Royal College of General Practitioners (1987) *If only I had the time*. Centre for Medical Learning, Dundee.

Royal College General Practitioners (1990) *Who killed Susan Thompson?* Video and course book. RCGP, London.

Royal College of General Practitioners (1992) *Interview assessment form*. Unpublished.

Royal College of General Practitioners (1992) *Can we talk?* Video and course book. RCGP, London.

Stewart R (1979) *The reality of management*. Pan, London.

Turner R (1992) The benefit of effective staff delegation. *Practice Manager*. 2, 17–18.

Turrill T (1986) *A Challenge for the NHS*. Institute of Health Service Managers, London.

Wilson J and Cole G (1990) A healthy approach to performance appraisal. *Personnel Management*. 6, 46–9.

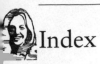

Index

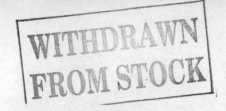